A Rainforest Asylum:
The enduring legacy of colonial psychiatric care in Malaysia

**Critical Studies
in Socio-Cultural Diversity**

Editor-in-Chief: Dr Sara Ashencaen Crabtree

Current and future titles in the same series

Practice Research in Nordic Social Work:
Knowledge production in transition
Edgar Marthinsen and Ilse Julkunen

The Cup, The Gun and The Crescent:
Social welfare and civil unrest in Muslim societies
Sara Ashencaen Crabtree, Jonathan Parker & Azlinda Azman

Active ageing?
Perspectives from Europe on a vaunted topic
María Luisa Gómez Jiménez, and Jonathan Parker (Editors)

Men and Masculinities in Europe (2nd edition)
Keith Pringle, Jeff Hearn, Harry Ferguson,Dimitar Kambourov,
Voldemar Kolga, Emmi Lattu, Ursula Müller, Marie Nordberg, Irina
Novikova,Elzbieta Oleksy, Joanna Rydzewska (Editors)

A Rainforest Asylum

The enduring legacy of colonial psychiatric care in Malaysia

Sara Ashencaen Crabtree

Whiting & Birch
MMXII

© Whiting & Birch Ltd 2012
Published by Whiting & Birch Ltd,
Forest Hill, London SE23 3HZ

ISBN 9781861771285

Printed in England and the United States by Lightning Source

With love and gratitude to those constant
lodestars by which my craft was steered:
Jonathan Parker, *mi alma gemela*
and Jack Crabtree, the Magus.

Contents

Preface

Probably when most people think of an ethnographic study of the people of East Malaysia, incorporating the two Malaysian states on the island of Borneo, they are more likely to think in terms of colourful cultural studies of indigenous folk struggling to maintain traditional lifestyles in the face of rampant industrialisation and consumerism. Or some equally emotive social issue such as this. Unsurprisingly, and fortunately, there are consequently many such noteworthy ethnographic accounts that chart change among rural communities in this region.

This study is somewhat different: in that although it focuses on the lives of certain Malaysian citizens of many ethnic backgrounds, pitted against what seems at times to be impersonal and oppressive forces, the context is far removed from the pastoral or the traditional. It is one, however, that has deep roots in Malaysian society and therefore forms the essential framework of this study.

These experiences have been gathered into a series of accounts from those individuals, who were then, and often still are, psychiatric patients living in long-term institutional care. The words of both sexes are encapsulated here; which is of particular importance as the narratives of psychiatric patients in Malaysia are rarely heard, and especially the voices of Malaysian women under this form of duress virtually unknown.

Significantly, it is argued that the context of Malaysian psychiatric institutional care is not inherently premised on indigenous needs and practices but is an uprooted, transplanted and anachronistic creation of another culture, from another time, for other purposes, based on assumptions and beliefs that have not survived intact from its own place of origin. Despite these anomalies however, the institution continues unscathed in Malaysia with no real sign of becoming obsolete or refashioned in this post-colonial nation despite the changes that are generally taking place in psychiatric services globally. Such paradoxes and the lived experiences of those patients accordingly form the theme of this book.

Acknowledgements

I have many people to thank on the long road towards the completion of this book, a large number of whom, being participants in this study, must sadly remain unnamed. However, those to whom I can give public thanks include my doctoral supervisor Dr Roger Green of the University of Hertfordshire, whose methodological incisiveness and acerbic wit served to pull me back onto the right track when faced with a jungle of enticing alternative paths. Many thanks also to Dr Lau Kim Kah who provided additional supervisory expertise and held the key to many an otherwise locked vault of hidden knowledge. Mick Bowman of the Sarawak Mental Health Association offered numerous invaluable insights into psychiatric care in the region. My long-suffering comrades Gabriel Chong and Dr Hew Cheng Sim ironed out logistical problems more than once with their practical know-how. My three final-year social work students Chan Soak Fong, Pek Wooi Ling and Jessing Ak Awos supplied able assistance through their professional translation skills and enthusiasm for the study. Thanks are additionally due to Dr Ann Appleton who kindly assisted me to update my knowledge in 2009 when other sources ran dry. Further thanks are due to Professor Shula Ramon in her capacity as critical friend. Finally, great debts of gratitude are owed to my late spouse and raconteur par excellence Professor Jack Crabtree for his consistent faith and keen editorial eye; and to my husband Professor Jonathan Parker for taking up the mantle of academic mentor, advisor and faithful helpmate. Finally, I would like to thank and commend my publisher David Whiting for all his advice and support.

I
Introduction

In 1996, fresh from university studies, I was delighted to leave a wintry Britain to take up my first academic post in Malaysia – a compellingly fascinating region. My first experience of Malaysia was the congested capital city of Kuala Lumpur, where bristling, hyper-modern skyscrapers towered over the more sedate, colonial villas and municipal landmarks, thus defying many of my more outdated notions of the city. Finally, I arrived in Sarawak, East Malaysia, which I found both beautiful and sufficiently steeped in a polymorphous and multifaceted heritage to satisfy my romantic instincts and where I lived very happily for the next five years. Settling in at the local university I subsequently learned probably as much from my friendly, multicultural Malaysian students as I taught them of the social sciences.

At some point during those first exciting, confusing and frenetic months of orientation I became aware of the existence of a discreetly located psychiatric hospital built some sixty or so years earlier. I had long been interested in mental health issues and resolved to learn more about mental health provision in this area at the first opportunity. As I settled into my new life, it became apparent that the hospital had been virtually untouched by previous external research, and yet appeared to offer an intriguing picture of post-colonial psychiatric care that invited closer attention.

After making some initial overtures to the hospital authorities, I was eventually sufficiently privileged to be permitted to carry out a series of research studies at the hospital, which for the purposes of confidentiality, whilst trying to remain true to the appellations of many psychiatric hospitals in Malaysia, I have duly called 'Hospital Tranquillity'. This book, the culmination of my research studies there, represents a pioneering experience for me in view of the dearth of research activities taking place on such topics regionally.

Moreover, the few studies undertaken on mental health issues in Malaysia have mostly been scientifically based. Therefore, being quantitative in methodology, they have not focused upon subjective experiences, particularly those of psychiatric patients, which incontestably formed a serious deficit in our understanding of mental health phenomena.

A gap in the literature, therefore, was evident. Thus the study, after duly negotiating logistical problems and the potential quagmires of ethics committees, commenced in 1997. Reaching a zenith in the new millennium, it was periodically dusted down in the intervening years. Now fully revived and revised, this ethnography offers an account of the lives of both patients and staff in a post-colonial psychiatric institution in Malaysia. In so doing it has drawn from a particularly influential well of knowledge – the surge of interest by historians in colonial psychiatry – which has illuminated many of the phenomena noted in this study; and which may be seen to make its own tangential contribution to our dislocated understandings of historically situated care.

*

The aim of the ethnographic approach, which is the chosen form of methodology used here, links the narratives of participants to the overarching theme relating to the embedded nature of the colonial paradigms of the asylum, which, it is argued, are implicitly enacted at Hospital Tranquillity. Ethnography enables the researcher to engage closely with a complex social situation. It is the pursuit of understanding of the 'culture' of the setting through an analysis of the conditions of individuals therein, premised upon and grounded in their experiences and perspectives. Accordingly, the concept of 'culture' defines how participants view their world, and interact with and from within it, using a phenomenological view. Here it serves to define the categories of participants: as 'patients' or 'staff' with implicit and explicit social guidelines that prescribe expected conduct for each group. Naturally, however, individuals frequently do not react or behave in the way that might be predicted from their acculturation (Helman, 1990). Consequently, the descriptions of participants across the institutional strata are noted in reference to their experiences of hospital life, albeit often from very different perspectives. The strong resonance between narratives and theory therefore seeks to lend a muscular and vigorous credibility to a critical discussion of postcolonial psychiatric services in contemporary Malaysia.

Furthermore, as will be discussed in more detail in Chapter Two, this study does not attempt to camouflage or obviate the mediating influences of my cultural background, but instead openly exploits this as a prism through which to interpret findings and my role as a researcher. My position as a British, white and female researcher therefore creates an interesting resonance in research undertaken in a developing country with a British colonial heritage, and is explored in greater depth.

Finally, I would add that, as this is a study of a unique phenomenon, it would be unwise to make gross generalisations across all psychiatric institutions in Malaysia or to assume that one psychiatric hospital is exactly the same as another (Brewer, 2000; Hammersley, 1990b). As will be seen however, the narratives of participants do raise important questions for contemporary services in this region, and serve to increase our awareness and comprehension of the development of mental health services in other postcolonial nations. Those services considered here are grounded in the historical context of colonialism in Malaya and its relationship with the advancing profession of psychiatry practised on subject nations. That many of these traditional, and often very oppressive, practices and attitudes can still be found in current service delivery is at least disquieting and demands closer scrutiny. Yet, the insights provided by analyses of colonial psychiatry suggest that there are some close parallels to be drawn in the evolutions of psychiatry between Malaysia and Britain in particular, and also across the other nations of the Commonwealth.

A guide to terms and semantics

After grappling with the ethics of what constitutes confidentiality issues in research and to whom or how this should be extended, as well as for whose interests, I have decided on a compromise in which both the names of all participants have been carefully disguised, as has the name of the hospital. The geographical location of the hospital is implied but not specified, as clarification of the role the hospital plays in the wider, multicultural community is essential to our understanding of its local and regional importance.

Furthermore, I regularly refer to people admitted to the hospital as 'patients' rather than using the more progressive and popular term 'service user'. This latter term has become ubiquitous in the UK, for example, where it is strongly associated with consumer choice towards psychiatric services (including the issue of the right to refusal of services). It emphasises individual rights and empowerment and stands in contrast to the more passive term of 'patient'. Therefore, my reasons for not using the term 'service user' are conscious and pointed, and first of all relate to the fact that primarily the term is in rare currency in Malaysia. It is also one that is not used by informants at the study site, and I consider it more in keeping with an ethnographic approach not to impose titles relating specifically to the context, but which are nonetheless unfamiliar to it. The term 'patient' by contrast is one generally utilised by parties employed, admitted or visiting the hospital, and is therefore the one I have adopted throughout this study.

In addition, the hospital is occasionally referred to as an 'asylum' by some participants. This term however carries very powerful connotations, as, for example, has been used to notable effect by Erving Goffman in describing the almost complete lack of autonomy characteristic of the 'total institution' in which all normal functions of life are carried out in a regimented fashion under a single supervisory authority (Goffman, 1991). Some of the findings discussed in the study depict institutional practices at Hospital Tranquillity, which are commensurate with Goffman's terminology and illustrative examples. I have therefore appropriated the term 'asylum' and use it in a deconstructive manner to describe certain aspects of hospital policy and episodes of patient care, which I feel comply rather more with a highly custodial and disempowering environment for patients and for staff, than with the practices compatible with Western contemporary consumer ideology. However, equally I recognise that the term 'asylum' also corresponds to the notion of a haven, which holds historical resonances to the establishment of such institutions, as explored in more detail in Chapter Three. Additionally, in Chapter Four, the first of the chapters on fieldwork, this tension is explored in more detail in relation to participant experiences of the psychiatric institution as both imprisoning and as acting as a refuge. Finally, in relation to the process of fieldwork, I refer to those interviewed as both 'respondent' and 'participant'. I am conscious that I use these terms according to subtle nuances, in that 'respondent' tends to indicate to me a more formalised interview relationship than that implied by the latter term. Nonetheless, for the reader's benefit I would conclude by saying that in effect these terms are used more or less synonymously.

The social and historical background to the study

The city where the study took place is relatively small and prosperous, with a largely white-collar workforce mainly employed in Government administration, served by a large population of shopkeepers and commercial workers (Hew, 1999). It is a rapidly changing city in a region long wealthy in natural resources, but these have been regularly exploited, causing the dispossession of many indigenous groups. For the most part the region's resources are harvested by the less well-off and comparatively over-populated Peninsula. This is not to say that the new opportunities and prosperity have not succeeded in filtering down to many people. Nonetheless, for the social scientist it is not necessary to be equipped for a lengthy expedition to find many examples of hard-core poverty, literally on the ample, polished doorstep of the city.

The Chinese presence in the city is evident, where streets are dominated by Chinese food outlets and ornamented by colourful Buddhist temples. However, the attempt to alter the Chinese ethnic flavour of the city is accelerating, where, for example, many of the old colonial street names of long dead British administrators, along with prominent ethnic Chinese personalities, are gradually being replaced with those that reinforce a focus on the country's prevailing power balance.

Briefly, the historical background to modern Malaysia effectively starts in 1957 when Malaya gained its independence from Britain. In 1963 the two States of East Malaysia, Sarawak and Sabah, joined with Malaya to form the Federation of Malaysia. Since then political lines have been drawn in the enshrinement of pro-discriminatory policies towards Malays and indigenous peoples in the country's constitution, whereby these groups are welded together under the title *bumiputera*, literally 'sons of the soil'.

The New Economic Policy in 1971 continues to be regarded as a contentious political strategy. As Cleary and Eaton (1992: 93) point out, 'positive discrimination …. has meant that there is considerable economic self-interest attached to classification methods'. This has fuelled, one might add, considerable resentment amongst non-*bumiputera* citizens, as well as proving an expensive expedient in many ways for the country as a whole (Kheng, 2003). Yet, it is also argued that even among the identified *bumiputera* inequalities exist between the 'birthright' Malay *bumiputera* and those among the indigenes who have acquired this status through religious conversion to Islam (Baba, 2010). Not surprisingly, the affirmative action policy was the basis of the conflict between the newly founded Malaysia and Chinese-dominated Singapore, resulting in the latter's expulsion from the Federation in 1965.

The effect of this is that the *bumiputera* have been able to purchase land at a favourable price in all areas. The Chinese and other non-indigenous groups, however, have not been allowed this latitude, and are concentrated in urban areas. This consequently has an influence on the demographic population of consumers of psychiatric services that are predominantly urban based, and which forms an important context to the discourses of patient 'race' or ethnicity, discussed at greater length in Chapter Eight.

Popularly psychiatric hospitals and asylums have often been regarded as deplorable institutions, redolent of abuse, neglect, abandonment and at best unmitigated tedium and rigid routine. In fiction Kesey's sensationalised novel *One Flew Over the Cuckoo's Nest* depicted medical treatment, specifically ECT (electro-convulsive therapy) as brutal, punitive and ultimately destructive of individual autonomy (Kesey, 1962). However, Goffman's (1968, 1991, 1993) far more sober, academic study also depicts the psychiatric institution as fundamentally dehumanising.

In some regions of the world, psychiatric services have supplied a notoriously poor service, such as, for example, the 'chaotic and miserable' environment of Greece's psychiatric community on the island of Leros (Strutti and Rauber, 1994: 309). This hit the headlines in the 1980s with photographs of naked, disorientated patients of indeterminate sex in many cases, being hosed down with cold water, like so much cattle, by indifferent and demoralised staff. Leros seemed to typify the worst conditions of asylum care of an earlier age and maybe even of other developing countries, as asserted in the following statement.

> Mental hospitals in the Third World are fairly dreadful places, and there are many in which custodial care is the only intention, ECT the usual treatment, staff brutality is commonplace, all patients compulsorily detained and few ever discharged (Rack, 1982: 171).

Large scale reform of psychiatric services have in fact taken place, such as that under Franco Basaglia, who spearheaded the attack on the abusive systems of psychiatric institutions in Europe, resulting in legal changes in Italy in the late seventies. While following on from this in latter years British service users, for instance, have succeeded in speaking out about the brutalities and repressions of institutional care (Laing, 1996; Sainsbury Centre for Mental Health, 1998).

Additionally, in the West a feminist body of critique has built up to explore the particular significance of psychiatry in relation to women service users. This argues that women are exposed in great numbers world-wide to a male-dominated medical hierarchy that replicates the patriarchal oppression of society within the stigmatising and controlling confines of psychiatric services (Chesler, 1996; Russell, 1995; Showalter, 1985). Although the United Nations have acknowledged that women suffer massively from the trauma of violence and oppression, little has specifically been written concerning the position of women in psychiatric services beyond the ethnocentric focus of the West although certainly this is a subject that deserves greater academic focus (Wetzel, 2000).

Consequently, in considering psychiatric care in developing regions, the condition of women is frequently subsumed by the generic plight of patients *per se*, rather than subjected to gender differentials. In this study, there has been an endeavour to amply the otherwise relatively muted voices of Malaysian women, predominantly, as patients; however, there has also been a concerted attempt to apply a gender-based analysis to the lives of psychiatric staff, both nurses and the rare female doctor as well.

Although psychiatry is a relatively new profession and, as can be seen, has been besmirched by negative stereotypes, the institutional environment in which psychiatry has been practiced has often been viewed with enormous social stigma accompanied by social anxieties. As argued here, the exporting of the asylum model to the colonies, such as colonial Malaya, did not appear to evolve a new approach to care, but merely engaged in transferring not only contemporary skills and knowledge of the time, but social attitudes as well. This then is the background to the study of the hospital which, being built at the end of the colonial era, has seen many changes in the care of psychiatric patients. It continues to be an important example of institutional responses to social and political developments towards mental illness and the welfare of those who use the services.

Organisation and navigation

The final section of this chapter seeks to assist the reader in their navigation of the text. Accordingly, *Chapter Two* focuses upon the use of ethnographic methodology and methods underpinning this study. The logistics of field work are additionally discussed in respect to the crucial forging of relationships with participants, and finally, ethical considerations in fieldwork.

Chapter Three critically scopes the literature devoted to the historical background of evolving psychiatric services in the West, colonial territories in the Indian subcontinent and elsewhere, and subsequently Malaya and Borneo.

The findings of the study commence in *Chapter Four*, by locating Hospital Tranquillity within a historical, geographical, social and cultural context. Following this, a discussion of the routines, rituals and the socialisation process of life in the ward environment is offered.

Chapter Five concentrates on the hierarchical socialisation of individuals and relationships between patients. This concludes with an examination of the nature and utilisation of patient labour structured on stereotypical gender divisions.

In *Chapter Six* methods of patient control are reviewed, such as treatment programmes that include electro-convulsive therapy. The chapter concludes with a 'service user' view of how medication is used at the hospital.

Subsequently *Chapter Seven* considers how women patients are subject to stringent control in terms of freedom of movement consistent with patriarchal stereotypic notions of gender and mental illness.

The following chapters are devoted to issues of staffing. The conditions of work at the hospital are considered in *Chapter Eight*, where professional practice and career opportunities are viewed against a backdrop of the national policy debate on service delivery. In *Chapter Nine*, staff strategies of control and containment of patients are explored, along with staff perceptions of risk and violence in working with psychiatric patients.

Finally, *Chapter Ten* draws the findings together in a concluding discussion.

2

Fieldwork and field relationships

Social science studies that engage directly with the issue of culture, both as conceptual and overlapping social construction, as well as 'culture' enacted as a unfamiliar and factual reality, such as is the case here, have typically been classified as essentially anthropological in essence. Classic anthropological ethnographies have almost invariably taken place in locations far removed from the home environment of the researcher, such as those of Malinowski in New Guinea (1922) or Mead in Samoa (1943). These locations have often been perceived as exotic or in some other sense removed from the familiar. Nancy Scheper-Hughes, for instance, leaves the United States of America and chooses rural Ireland, which appears to represent a sharp contrast to her own cultural background; subsequently writing an account of anomie, social and, arguably, cultural stagnation and mental illness (Scheper-Hughes, 1982). Sue Estroff, by contrast, emphasises that her ethnographic study of mental illness in Wisconsin takes place in her own hometown. Although this was a study from home, she conveys the polarisation between the underground existence of a deeply marginalised group of people and the privileges of the comfortable, conventional living standards that she is familiar with (Estroff, 1985). Scheper-Hughes also offered an account of neonatal mortality in impoverished communities in Brazil. This locates the mature author as a foreigner from the First World, but whose association with the country and rationale for research has been formed through the influences of a period of residence there as a young voluntary worker (Scheper-Hughes, 1992).

My own particular situation approximates in some ways to that of Scheper-Hughes in the latter example, in that Malaysia was my home for some years. This resulted in my ambivalent position of being both familiar with, as well as being a stranger to, the region. My status, however, was that of a non-permanent resident with no citizen rights and subject to the terms of temporary employment. I was therefore only partially assimilated with tenuous ties and commitments, which I was aware would begin to atrophy with my departure. The identification I felt were filtered through the conditions of being a foreign alien; and therefore, as John Clammer (1987) notes, my fieldwork experiences were mediated through layers of belonging, with all the associate problems of immersion in a new cultural context . Nonetheless, I would not claim that this work belongs exclusively to the anthropological oeuvre, although it resonates with that discipline as much as it does with medical sociology. Perhaps its best defence is to claim the exciting territory of the fault line between the two, as well as drawing inspiration and illumination from psychiatric historiography, and accordingly it stands unapologetically as a robust and painstaking interdisciplinary study.

The research process

In terms of the methodology underpinning this study, ethnography, once the preserve of anthropologists, this has been adopted across a range of social science disciplines, and beyond. It is arguably the method par excellence for undertaking an in-depth inquiry into the otherwise esoteric world of 'cultures', to use the term once more in its wider sociological meaning. Commensurately, the aim of ethnography, is, as van Maanen (1988: 4) pithily suggests, to 'decode one culture while recording it for another'. Furthermore, much has been written about ethnography as both a methodology and a method of data collection, a large corpus of which has been published as guidance for the novice researcher, as well as making an important contribution to philosophies of knowledge. Accordingly, this well trodden path will not be revisited here in any detail. Suffice to say, therefore, that the bulk of data collection took place over a sixteen-month period, reaching a culmination in 2000, with periodic updates taking place up to 2009.

During the intensive data collection period dozens of interviews took place with both patients and staff, as well as other prominent mental health service providers, together with some focus group discussions held in the hospital and at a 'halfway home': a community-based supported lodging scheme for ex-patients. Interviewing methods varied in type and style depending upon my participants and the circumstances – from in-depth but unstructured, individual or group discussions to intensive semi-structured, recorded interviews. Other data collection methods that I commonly used included critical observation and the use of statistical records from the hospital archives. The utilisation of all these different methods, typical of the flexible ethnographic approach, ensured a degree of triangulation against which to test my findings and developing hypotheses.

So much for methods, which were embedded in established ethnographic technique. In relation to methodology, ethnography naturally stands as a form of epistemology where, in keeping with its postmodernist, relativistic roots, one evolutionary branch has given rise to 'critical ethnography'. This is fundamentally emancipatory in its general aims, and seeks to make the necessary links between the narratives and lives of participants and the structural constraints of wider society, in relation to issues of disenfranchisement and disempowerment of the individual (DeLaine, 1997). Emancipatory ethnography, therefore, is overtly embedded in what Ortner (1995: 173) describes as an enterprise of 'intellectual and moral positionality', and this formed the bedrock for my work. However, it is also one where, like *generic* ethnography, for want of a better expression, a critical scrutiny of a wider audience beyond the researcher is needed to evaluate how rigorously and scrupulously research has been carried out and conclusions drawn. To this end, ethnographers need to take into account that they are necessarily part of the social study and cannot be omitted from their accounts (Hammersley and Atkinson, 2010).

Consequently, gender issues are closely considered here, where the experiences of men have been used for comparative purposes with those of women (Stanley and Wise, 1993). This inclusion avoids distortion of a phenomenon that is shared in multiple ways by men and women patient participants at the hospital, but also permits points of difference to emerge. An attempt has been made to seek an understanding of the lives of 'patients' as they are informed by gender and this acts as an important but not exclusive category of analysis, forming what Sandra Harding refers to as the 'problematics' of the study (Harding, 1987: 30).

The construction of any ethnography, however, does not stand on findings alone, but is viewed as the subjection of data to a process of 'textualisation'. Here, to utilise van Maanen's (1988: 95) definition, data are subjected to the process of atomisation and classification, where they are sifted and reorganised through analysis (Aunger, 1995: 97). As Hammersley and Atkinson observe:

> It is now widely recognised that 'the ethnography' is produced as much by how we write as by the processes of data collection and analysis (Hammersley and Atkinson, 1993: 239).

However, as van Maanen (1988: 1) and Ortner (1995) argue, for the researcher the ethnographic process equally involves serious moral responsibility, particularly in relation to the representation of phenomena and participants. This counters the typical stance of classical ethnography where the influence of the researcher upon the study was fundamentally discounted in the text. This Olympian stance has subsequently raised contentious issues regarding the validity of ethnographic accounts, which have in turn served to raise some very fruitful debates and the development of new epistemological strategies.

The question of whether this particular study offers a truthful account of lives can be viewed from at least two points of view. Firstly, as Berg states, ethnography is an inexact science whereby hypotheses can be evaluated in terms of *plausibility* but not in terms of *validity* (Berg, 2007). As the reliability of the theory can be evaluated *prima facie* by the frequency of similar occurrences noted within categories, the critical reader might conclude that it is not unreasonable to accept *this* particular theory based on *these* particular observations (Hammersley, 1990b). Furthermore (self) reflexivity, therefore acts as a form of epistemology that serves to make the ontological 'social' world that exists independently of us, known (Aull Davies, 1999: 17).

Associated with issues of objectivity, the representation of the accounts of participants raises other issues. Linda Alcott (1991: 6-7) points out that the social location of the speaker affects the 'meaning and truth' of what is said, in addition to the concealed dangers inherent in speaking on behalf of less privileged groups. The discursive problematics of speaking *for* and speaking *about* are brought to the foreground, where the latter can be dangerously conflated with the former. All, however, is not lost, a way forward is proposed:

> It *is* possible (and indeed desirable) to speak of 'others' but only when the reader can clearly see where the speaker is 'coming from'. Autobiography (read as self-identification) becomes the basis upon which white feminists authenticate speech, such that *failure* to identify speaker location is potentially racist and classist and sexist. While the act of 'identification' may precede equally oppressive practices, it nonetheless signals a more 'honest' beginning (Lyons, 1999: 6).

What Lyons (1999), following Aull Davies (1999) is proposing therefore is a methodological stance grounded in self-reflexivity, whereby the focus revolves around the location of the speaker. In this study self-reflexivity also pivots around the issue of accountability and emancipatory goals, as well as clarity. Accordingly, the specific properties of gender, ethnicity and class, for instance, that characterise the researcher are considered, as inherently forming a personal/political/cultural lens through which the phenomena is studied, and of which the reader should be rightly be aware (Burman, 1999).

> Thus the researcher appears in these analyses not as an invisible, anonymous, disembodied voice of authority, but as a real, historical individual with concrete, specific desires and interests – and ones that are sometimes in tension with each other (Harding, 1987: 32).

Self-reflexivity, therefore, creates a space in which a critique of authorship, authority and cultural representation can be constructed (Hirsch and Olson, 1995). Despite the scepticism of critiques, such as that offered by Patai (1991) the self-reflexive strategy effectively responds to a question posed by Pettman, of how 'dominant group women address their whiteness' in relation to cultural difference, a question germane to this study in relation to the postcolonial context of research and my own cultural heritage (Pettman, 1992: 155). Self-reflexivity therefore creates a legitimate way of addressing how neo-colonialism in developing regions impact upon 'First World' researchers – an issue especially germane to this study (Visweswaran, 1988).

Before leaving the topic of research methods altogether, a brief explanation of the process of data analysis is advisable. In ethnography data analysis does not occupy the discrete, hygienic position of analytic processes in the hard sciences, but runs parallel and continuously alongside data collection. This permits the researcher to thereby change tack in a timely fashion: abandoning paths that have led to barren cul-de-sacs, while pursuing more fruitful ones. Typically, therefore in my own research, daily observations and interviews were noted by hand and coded by computer-aided software into single instances or recurring ones that were later developed into themes (Brewer, 2000; Tesch, 1991). Once no further patterns emerge from the study, saturation has been reached and data collection can be completed. The next step is normally withdrawal from the study site – by no means, an easy process, due to the difficult human elements of being obliged to dismantle edifices of close contact, arduously built up in the interests of creating good, and often quite intimate relationships with participants, as will be further discussed in Chapter Ten.

Gatekeepers and participants

Hospital Tranquillity stands in a certain amount of isolation compared to policy developments, funding and political focus, which are concentrated in Peninsular Malaysia, despite it being an important regional resource. Currently the hospital is facing the dilemma of how to address the practicalities of ideological developments in health care within the context of contemporary political debate in Malaysia. This in turn represents significant challenges for the future direction of the hospital and its community services - critical issues that were revisited in conversations with staff on several occasions during the fieldwork process.

In commencing fieldwork permission was initially sought from the *Jabatan Kesihatan Negeri X* (the State Department of Health), but it was the Director's personal consent as the main gatekeeper that would prove crucial for work to proceed. I am doubtful whether my position as a foreigner actually assisted in the facilitation of this process of consent, as Punch (1993) discovered in his study of an Amsterdam police force, although it is clear that my status as a local lecturer was quite definitely helpful. Fortunately the Director of the hospital, Dr T.W., was already known to me from my previous research projects, and furthermore we both served on the committee of a local mental health NGO (non-governmental organisation). Burgess describes how an attempt to return to a previous field site for further studies was not welcomed by the principal gatekeeper (Burgess, 1991). By contrast, in my own case I found that the Director was amenable to further work at the hospital, since familiarity with my prior activities worked in my favour, and proved to be very valuable in allaying concerns about my integrity and ability as a researcher.

This alliance proved to be extremely helpful on numerous occasions in smoothing the path of obstacles in relation to access to wards and interviews. In his role as the main gatekeeper of the site, Dr T.W. was in a position to grant a general consent on behalf of his staff, and to a large extent in practical terms those of his patients as well. This proved to be less helpful than I anticipated in terms of ethics and practical assistance. Roger Homan for instance raises issue with the ethics of such generalised consent, the right of consent by, for instance, individual staff members is effectively withheld (Homan, 1991). Pragmatically Burgess points out that even where the consent of main gatekeepers is obtained this does not remove the need to negotiate terms with individual staff informants as informal gatekeepers who may otherwise provide blocks to adequate research (Burgess, 1995).

Naturally, responses to participation varied, many patients expressed positive opinions, although others were clearly quite indifferent to my reasons, but just welcomed the chance for a chat with an outsider. A small minority rejected my advances outright and in keeping with the experiences of other ethnographers, some participants became close allies and main contributors of insider knowledge (Glick, 1998: Punch, 1993). After all my precautions regarding confidentiality and consent I was fairly surprised at first that few patients seemed particularly bothered by this. More important to most patients on the ward was my ability to keep a secret when it came to whispered confidences about a particular 'scam' or an incident of abusive behaviour from a certain member of staff.

Gaining consent for interviews with individual patients did not completely ensure a smooth passage to fieldwork and here problems were threefold. First of all the director's consent was generally broadcast via a memorandum that apparently was not circulated to all members of staff, and therefore my presence needed to be explained, clarified and re-checked on numerous occasions throughout the field-study period. It was quite common for my credentials to be inquired into time and again, and occasionally pointed inquiries were made about whether the Dr T.W.'s permission had *really* been granted.

Secondly, this form of generalised consent from a superior did not necessarily guarantee willing participation from respondents, exemplifying the simple observation by Miles and Huberman, that 'weak consent leads to poorer data' (1994: 291). This could additionally be seen when initially, in a bid to be helpful, some members of staff tried to coerce patients into cooperating with me. Although I quickly discouraged such practices, I was also aware of a possible double game being played by staff, in that this could also act as an effective strategy of diversion away from them.

Finally, and connected to the point of weak consent, despite the director's consent, it was nonetheless quite difficult to engage in a further process of negotiation with staff members acting as 'gatekeepers' to their wards. I often found that staff were reluctant to discuss terms with me and seemed to prefer this to be confined to my discussions with the director, and then mandated by him. This seemed to be particularly true of female nursing members of staff and junior male counterparts, both groups sharing a common and lowlier status in the medical hierarchy. Yet by not being able to negotiate openly with members of staff, I felt that their concerns were not specifically addressed, and frequently I perceived their unspoken or indirectly conveyed resentment and anxiety about my research role. I was regularly directed to talk to a more senior member of staff in corresponding male or female wards, under the pretext that this person was a more knowledgeable and experienced individual. In reality a formal repository of professional knowledge was usually not the best informant, as in this role such individuals tended to deliver set pieces of information concerning policies governing the management of the hospital that rarely provided useful insights into the lived experience. Instead it seemed to be that this role was largely a symbolic one designed to keep parties from the outside at bay, as well as providing the authority to speak, so clearly lacking among many women workers and inexperienced younger men.

Unfortunately, I found that discomfort and hostility towards my presence on the ward were not uncommon features of fieldwork. Like Van Maanen I did on occasions experience something approaching 'unambiguous rejection', although not as bluntly expressed as his examples quoted from hard-bitten New York cops (Van Maanen, 1991: 36-7). On one occasion Sister Magdalene, a senior member of staff, audibly instructed a subordinate to inform me that she was far too busy to talk to me when, so far as I could see, the ward was very quiet and she did not seem to be specifically engaged in work. It should be noted that this conversation took place within a few feet of where I was standing and delivered in a tone of annoyed dismissal, to be subsequently delivered in evident embarrassment by the auxiliary nurse. Two further examples taken from my field notes illustrate this rejection; the first takes place in an episode on Male Ward 1 where, as usual, a patient is helping two medical assistants with medication to be dispensed to patients on the locked section.

Field notes. Male Ward 1:

Ahi, a Malay MA (Medical Assistant) turned up (he's not too friendly towards me most of the time) just as I was writing down the patient audit from the nursing chart. He starts helping Bong to hand out medication to the locked section with Hui Ling helping. As usual I am surprised by how compliant and passive people are when they take their meds. One poor man in the open section keeps asking to go back home in Malay: '*balik kampung, bila?*' (When do I go home to my village?). The MAs ignore him. He then appeals to me, maybe because I am White and possibly influential, to take him back to his remote Iban kampung in X. Bong, another patient, helps with translation.

Bong: He says that he has had ECT so now wants to go back home.
Researcher: Has it helped him?

Bong:	Yes, he is much more stable now. [To Ahi] How many more?
Ahi:	Three more, course of six.

While I am taking to Bong a patient in the locked section is hanging around the grill and talking incessantly, non-stop and apparently unintelligibly. After some time of this I comment on it to Bong.

Researcher:	This must be hard for people to cope with.
Ahi:	[overhearing] That's why he is here. He talks all through the night. The brother says it drives them 'up the wall'. Non-stop talking, the words don't hang together though. [Pause] He talks so much he should get a job as a lecturer.
Researcher:	Yes, he'd be perfect - all he'd have to do is make sense.

[Ahi gives me a sly, side-look and laughs. Later as I am leaving]

Researcher:	Well, I must go now.
Ahi:	I hope this is worth your time.
Researcher:	I know it seems strange.
Ahi:	Yes.
Researcher:	But it is very interesting ... you learn a lot by observing.

This interaction with Ahi is a typical encounter representative of our relationship, in which in the space of a couple of hours he manages to get in two digs, the first conveying that I talk so much rubbish that I am no different from a particularly incoherent psychiatric patient. The second that I am wasting my time just hanging around watching the staff and no doubt, the message is also that I am wasting their time as well. Not surprisingly I never enjoyed spending time on the ward when Ahi was present, as I usually found myself in the position of trying to observe the ward while wincing at the pinpricks he delivered - when he was willing to acknowledge my presence at all. The second extract from my field notes highlights the difficulties of gathering data while in a state of awkward discomfort at being pointedly ignored by members of staff.

Field notes. Female Ward 2:

I wanted to follow up with the nurses on incidents of violence but was unable to get far. The staff sister, a handsome Iban woman, didn't seem at all pleased to see me despite a polite but frozen half-smile and made no attempt to talk to me or make me feel welcome. She sat with her back to me the whole time and ignored me throughout. After a while of this I went out onto the veranda to strike up conversation but the other two nurses seemed unwilling or unable to talk to me (perhaps they felt the bad vibes from the sister in charge or maybe their English wasn't up to it). These incidents made to feel unwelcome, to say the least!

I see this as all part-and-parcel of the research process and in fact research does act as both a wonderfully protective umbrella when it comes to all this negative grist to the mill. Yet there is a human dimension to all this, which I feel and is not easily shrugged off - it is this aspect in part which makes going into the field, an uncomfortable, anxiety-making business where you feel vulnerable, inquisitive - rarely wise and often foolish - an ambivalent position of unwelcome visitor and anticipated guest. As usual I often feel far more accepted by the patients than by the staff, today some seemed mildly interested and even pleased to see me.

Despite the general consent by the director to fieldwork, these examples clearly show the power held by informal gatekeepers to enable or block research activities through fairly simple but highly effective human strategies. Whilst of course, as Shaffir (1991) notes, knowing that this provides useful and additional insights for research, the discomfort generated by being made to feel something approaching a pariah acts as a significant handicap that needs to be constantly addressed and overcome. Through episodes like these I became deeply familiar with the almost ever present and heart-sinking sensations Van Maanen aptly refers to as caused by the 'stigma of the research role' (Van Maanen, 1991: 32).

I do not think that this feeling of stigma ever quite disappeared; and the discomfort and embarrassment of imposing myself in situations, where sometimes my welcome was qualified by many interwoven issues from many directions. All this made fieldwork fraught with nuance and expectations from patient and staff participants that often left me uncertain and anxious. Overt rejection from participants, such as the day I was spat upon by a patient, did not lower my spirits over much on reflection. More worrying was the feeling of guilt, helplessness and loss of control in the face of so much pathos and so many direct appeals for my help, my understanding or my allegiance, according to the agenda of my interlocutor. My own attitude to fieldwork was therefore often ambivalent, and there were days when only stringent self-discipline drove me forward, regardless of how experience had shown me I might feel by the end of a working day in the field, sometimes elated, satisfied, angry or depressed.

Planning the research campaign

Having formulated my research focus the next step was to consider how to study the institution. After due consideration I decided to concentrate primarily on four wards: two acute and two long-stay wards. Of these four wards, two were allocated to female and two to male patients; the latter were used to provide comparison for the purposes of my study. The long-stay wards and the private wards were used for orientation and comparative purposes and, along with the occupational therapy department, were visited many times. This department provided some relief from the wards, where I gained some extremely useful insights into gender stereotyping and patient labour. Finally, other wards such as the forensic ward, *Bunga Raya*, a floral epithet for a ward exclusively for male offenders, attracted my interest as did, although to a lesser extent, the sick ward.

The acute wards, Female Ward 1 and Male Ward 1, and the long-stay wards, Female Ward 2 and Male Ward 2, were chosen on the basis of a combination of factors. The acute wards provided an interesting basis for comparison with the long-stay wards, in view of the fact that the selected long-stay wards were not exclusively but generally more likely to be the eventual destination of acute patients later perceived to be chronically afflicted. The daily routines, recreation and patient and staff interactions were livelier on the acute wards with the exception of the forensic ward. On the wards selected most of the patients enjoyed comparative youth compared with the remainder of the long-stay wards; and therefore, to generalise, were more likely to be able to communicate with me as opposed to wards where there were a greater number of elderly and mentally infirm patients.

Overt observation techniques provided the major part of the data I gathered in which I made no pretence to on-lookers to be there for any other purpose than that of observation. This strategy conformed closely with that described by Tim May (1999: 140) in which the 'participant as observer' role is a public one. This involves not only observation but also the development of working relationships with participants as informants for the study. Information duly gathered in this way proved sufficient to obtain good insights into particularly interesting phenomena, such as methods of control or the use of patient labour on the wards. This also enabled me to make an informed decision regarding which wards should eventually be selected for closer scrutiny, as well as drawing my attention to those individuals whom I felt I could approach and those who might represent a threat to the study, or more prosaically, to myself.

In the early days, however, my method of observation was closer to that of a 'shotgun' approach in which interesting people, events and activities were noted down with little discrimination and less understanding, in a small, handy notebook on site. As the study progressed my comprehension of events taking place around me increased and allowed me to target certain phenomena on the ward. Patient mealtimes, medication routines, bedtimes and awakenings were just some of the events I sought to observe at certain times of the day and night. I therefore made myself present for early morning breakfast rounds on the wards, and mid-morning snacks; present for soporific afternoons and patient siesta time, and occasionally kept a night-time vigil with the staff night shifts. These latter shifts proved to be the most sociable and companionable, with staff most amused by my persistence and supportive of my endurance. On these occasions I could rely on coffee and *mee goring* (fried noodles) to be liberally supplied to keep tired eyes open, including mine.

At first, I had felt grotesquely conspicuous on the wards and felt that staff in varying degrees were self-conscious when going about their everyday business under these artificial circumstances. After a considerable amount of time and personal discomfort had lapsed I eventually manage to achieve a certain level of invisibility where everyone, staff and patients alike, apparently ignored my presence albeit on brief occasions. These occasions were punctuated by activities in which individuals would regularly engage me in conversations. Over time my explanations that I wanted to see what it was like on the wards began to be accepted by participants with less suspicion as to my exact motives.

In this way, therefore my observations narrowed down over time from a broad sweep of noting everything and anything that caught my attention to a narrow, and hopefully, more acute focus (Bannister, 1999). Through the use of observation techniques employed in a comparative exercise, I found that data from observations both informed and synthesised my developing hypotheses in a rigorous and synergistic relationship (Burgess, 1995).

Observation strategies on the wards allowed me freedom to adjust to situations taking place and consequently I would often engage or be approached by patient and staff informants. In common with Shaffir's (1991) experiences, most of these were informal conversations on a particular topic that I wanted to explore further. These interviews being 'unstructured' and 'flexible', informants often initiated the conversation from the outset (Lee, 1993). Here my interviewing strategy tended towards a deconstructive manoeuvre of attempting to uncover hierarchal distinctions through an appearance that was casual, with informal language and mannerisms, and generally trying to avoid with varying degrees of success the attitude and appearance of an *orang puteh* (White) lady visitor. Conversations with patients were fluid and spontaneous with participants joining in and departing from the discussion at hand as they pleased. This less formalised approach meant that patients chose the location to discuss matters and involved various settings. Occasionally we sat on stools under trees, or on the open veranda that most wards had, sometimes in the canteen or otherwise just sitting on beds inside the ward or in the rather bare recreation room. Some conversations took place in the occupational therapy department with patients chatting to me while they worked. Sometimes patients, usually men, would approach me to ask for a cigarette, which I did not have, or money, which I concealed, and then following this overture a discussion might be struck up. Similarly casual conversations with staff took place at the nursing station on wards, in private offices during tea breaks or while carrying out duties.

At other times, interviews were more formal when I wanted to discuss a range of issues based on a semi-structured interview guide that I had prepared earlier. The only criteria used for these interviews with patients were that they were willing to talk to me and fit enough to be interviewed; and here I relied on advice from the ward staff on the patient's state of health and lucidity. Semi-structured interviews with patients, as opposed to informal discussions, took place in the treatment room at the end of the wards. This room was separated from the main ward by a grill gate and was about the only private place that could be allocated to me. Nonetheless, interviews were often inadvertently interrupted by the nursing staff, cleaners or other patients who wandered in. Interviews would then be momentarily suspended if possible, before continuing. Semi-structured interviews were conducted at various intervals with selected members of staff, including medical officers, nursing staff and allied personnel, such as occupational therapists and the two social workers, as well as former members of staff. Normally these interviews required careful planning due to medical schedules and outpatient appointments, therefore they were usually tape-recorded and supplemented by extensive note taking during the interview process itself.

Semi-structured interviews with patients were usually taped with their consent. The open use of a tape recorder in informal situations was eventually seen to be too intrusive for general conversations after I detected that, in particular, members of staff felt uncomfortable and inhibited by the idea. Furthermore, I had the impression that the tape recorder was distracting for patients, as well as intrusive, and tended to curtail spontaneous disclosures. Reliance on an increasingly elastic memory for informal conversations meant the flow of conversation was not interrupted; and a more relaxed and confiding atmosphere could be created. Hastily but discreetly written up notes in shorthand on small notebooks usually took place in secluded corners of the ward following these valuable sessions, as like the patients I was not able to enjoy freedom of movement due to ward 'lock-up' procedures.

Although I had initially hoped to engage a wide range of respondents, in reality some were considerably more responsive than others. Opportunities to talk to both patients and staff were seized more on the basis of luck than design, commensurate with Burgess' definition of 'opportunistic sampling' (1995: 55).

Amongst the patient population my key informants were nearly all women; male patients tended to shy away from contact or at any rate often seemed less likely to respond to my questions with relevant information. On the face of it this is in keeping with the rapport Ann Oakley discovers in her research activities through the democratisation of the interviewing process, premised on the notion of shared commonalities, of which she writes:

> The women were reacting to my own evident wish for a relatively intimate and non-hierarchical relationship (Oakley, 1984: 47).

However, I lacked the basic common grounds that Oakley held; she was a British mother, interviewing British mothers. Whereas I was a foreign woman who had never been admitted to a psychiatric hospital and was attempting to develop a rapport with women and men, many of whom had spent years of their lives being processed by the Malaysian psychiatric services. Yet, despite Daphne Patai's (1991) critique of pseudo-identification, I remain convinced on my part that empathy of sorts was created during these times, albeit fractured with misunderstandings, cultural, social and sexual dissonances. Female patients in particular were often very friendly and even affectionate to varying degrees. I was subjected to a lot of gentle physical contact, and complimented, while at least one woman attempted to develop greater intimacy with me through sexual overtures.

The enveloping, cordial, affectionate and sometimes cloying atmosphere on the female wards was not replicated on the male wards. Rachel Forrester-Jones (1995) in reference to Ann Oakley, discusses the problem of creating reciprocal relationships with informants of the opposite sex to the researcher. Here, as Bailey (1996) notes, heterosexual and gender issues permeate the platonic boundaries of the relationship. Attempts at reciprocity are jeopardised by unshared gender expectations and politics, where women researchers may face the possibility of unwanted sexual advances from male participants. Accordingly, Estroff discusses the difficulties of negotiating relationships with male psychiatric informants whose social unfamiliarity with women creates a potential for painful misunderstandings.

> Being female helped and hurt. Over half of the subjects were men. My gender served as an entrée to contacting them and eliciting some interest, but it created tensions as well. Many had never had a female friend, that is, a symmetrical, platonic, heterosexual relationship. This led to some confusion of their part when their sexual advances offended me, and to reluctance on my part in entertaining situations with them that might be misconstrued. It was often inappropriate to participate with the group as the only female, and as a sexually inaccessible one, at that (Estroff, 1985: xvii).

Unlike Estroff's case, my contact with male patients did not take place in the social context of the community, but with only one exception, took place on the ward and for the most part in full sight of other patients and staff. Nevertheless, it was awkward and embarrassing to be the regularly subjected to so much inquisitive, blatant or wistful and forlorn attention from male patients, such as dealing with those who persisted in calling, flirting and chatting to me through the bars of the locked section. I was of course very aware that I was ultimately free to stay or go and they were confined, bored and excited by any break in the tedium, which by my presence I had caused. By persisting in staying on the ward, as fieldwork demanded, I was aware that I was also guilty of encouraging and exacerbating this mortifying sexual attention in an atmosphere of palpable, claustrophobic voyeurism. This verged, as Gearing (1995) found in relation to her own study, on sexual harassment. Furthermore, evasive strategies could not be properly mobilised, such as the feigned dignified, and casual indifference of a woman passing a building site, as this directly conflicted with the research guise of keen-eyed vigilance to detail. For the most part therefore, I tried to encourage relationships with male patients that were polite, friendly and neutral, in an atmosphere where physical contact and verbal intimacy were subtly discouraged. Obviously, there were exceptions to the rule, whereby some of my relationships with male patients were mutually respectful with no hint of a sexual overture on any occasion.

Contact with staff provided a fascinating contrast, in that, as stated, while female nursing staff were often reticent, their male counterparts - the 'medical assistants' - on the male wards were much more willing to disclose information to me than the female nursing staff and could be, when they chose to be, cheerful, amusing and friendly in their interactions with me. Such was the peculiar and intriguing balance in that in general women patients and male nursing staff were by far the most helpful and friendly towards me, whilst male patients and female nursing staff were often distant, close-lipped and occasionally overtly suspicious of me. As others have noted, women as researchers are seen as more harmless (and usually less socially important) than male researchers by male participants and therefore as less likely to use information in a damaging way (Gurney, 1991; Warren, 1988).

Any perceived lack of status on the grounds of gender may therefore have worked against forming a good rapport with female staff, in that there were few incentives for them to overcome the insider/outsider power dichotomy in an environment of closed ranks. Furthermore, Taylor (1991) points out that in his own research in a male-dominated setting rapport with informants was built upon a foundation of male solidarity, socialising activities and initiation ceremonies, something from which I was culturally barred in my own research with men and which did not materialise with women members of staff. Yet a few friendships were developed between myself and female members of staff, where one nurse occasionally pressed on me bottles of homemade *tuak* (rice wine), which at first I thought I was expected to pay for and only later realised were spontaneous gifts.

The conditioning of women to cautiously observe the boundaries between the sexes will continue to mediate relations in a research encounter. These will qualify the nature and depth of disclosures by informants as well as altering the agenda of what can be discussed in comparative safety for informants and researchers alike. I was, for example, very interested in learning more about the sexuality of male patients but this proved to be a problematic area for inquiry, and one where responses from male staff and patients were unsatisfactory, superficial and laden with implications. Lesbianism, however, was a subject that could be discussed with women, once relationships of comparative trust had been satisfactorily built. Reciprocity therefore is heavily dependent on gender relations in the field and consequently influences the quality of disclosures from informants. Like Forrester-Jones (1995) I feel that a male co-worker would have been able to elicit information from male informants that was to some degree inaccessible to me as a woman researcher in the field.

In his ethnographic account of psychiatric patients in Australia, Barrett (1996) makes full use of medical records and attends team meetings to augment information on informants. However, at an early stage of research I decided that I would not request access to patients' medical records although did note verbal information on patients from staff. My reasons were partially practical and partially ideological. Medical notes were kept on the ward and staff consultations of them took place in plain sight of patients, so that it was not possible to avoid being seen reading them. Any such activity would have been conspicuous and instantly noted by patients, and I feared that this therefore might interfere in forming relationships of trust with patients. Furthermore, I felt that these could probably contribute little in the way of understanding interactions in the hospital; my interest was located in everyday events and the perceptions of informants, rather than in turgid medical information, which could largely provide me only with details of admissions, discharges and medication. Finally, I also felt strongly that this was a transgression of privacy, to which my status as researcher could not really entitle me. This position was justified when patients prefaced their interviews by asking me if I had read their medical notes. I felt that my reassurance that I had not read them created a more confiding environment in which to seek personal disclosures from patients, who might otherwise see me as a sort of member of staff, or some such similar type of authority, although this of course did nevertheless happen.

Despite my good intentions however, I had not bargained for the frequent invitations by staff to read the notes. The nurses and medical assistants often seemed to feel the need to fit me into some type of legitimate medical role and offered me the records on numerous occasions, sometimes opening them at certain pages and putting them in front of me, which made it difficult to refuse a quick perusal. This bears comparison with Burgess's (1995) research experiences in a school setting, where he describes a similar need by staff to try and neutralise him through assimilation into the professional corps he was in part studying. Similarly therefore the invitation of medical notes not only legitimised my presence but also my research, which otherwise probably seemed a nebulous and unscientific way of going about things. The notes offered concrete and valid information in the eyes of staff, as opposed to the naïve and no doubt foolish questions I asked. My insistence on sitting with and talking to patients was commented on, to reiterate, with levity, incomprehension, or thinly veiled hostility.

Language and meaning

Competence in the language of informants is usually perceived to be part of the 'mystique' of ethnographic work, to paraphrase Aull Davies (1999: 76) who goes on to expand on the limitations imposed by reliance on translation. Accordingly, Agar (1996) comments on the uncomfortable feeling associated with having insufficient control during fieldwork when obliged to use interpreters, but comments that this is probably not an uncommon sensation for fellow researchers. Equally Ardener (1995: 106) notes how 'alienating' it can be to rely on translators and that time spent attempting to learn the language is well used. Martha Macintyre (1993) comments ruefully on the anthropological assumption of linguistic competence and her initial despair at her complete inability to speak Tubetube.

In East Malaysia, as in Peninsular Malaysia, the national language is Bahasa Malayu, and all Malaysian civil servants, including medical staff, are expected, in theory, to reach a high level of proficiency if they wish to secure permanent posts. The Peninsula uses a refined version, but in East Malaysia a shortened, simplified version is the common argot. This is not to suggest, however, that Bahasa Malayu is understood and used by everyone: the cultural diversity of people has meant that for many it remains a largely foreign tongue. The Dayak language Iban, for instance, has many similarities to Bahasa Malayu, but Bidayuh has a completely different structure and many obscure dialects. It is not uncommon to find that the older generation, specifically Chinese, Indian and Dayak families, speak English with greater fluency (due to the region's colonial history) than the official language. In the early sixties Dr K.E. Schmidt, described the problems caused by linguistic diversity in the following way:

> The chaos of languages in Sarawak constitutes the main difficulty for anyone concerned with mental health in this country. Among its bare three-quarters of a million people, at least twenty-one different languages (not dialects) are spoken. This situation obviously militates strongly against hospitalization, which is avoided as much as possible, since even normal people are unable to converse freely with each other (Schmidt, 1964:155).

At Hospital Tranquillity therefore a combination of languages and dialects are used, but most members of staff are familiar with English having been trained in that medium. Few patients, however, are particularly competent in English and will instead use a mixture of Malay, Iban,

Bidayuh and Chinese dialects, such as Foochow or Hokkien. Despite the plurality of languages, staff and patients manage to verbally interact reasonably well, and there is usually someone to hand who can translate.

As with Dr Schmidt, communication in my basic Malay was at first problematic, especially as my ability with other commonly used languages was non-existent. Painfully aware of my ineptness in this area I was happy to recruit a few of my most promising multilingual final-year social work students as translators some of the time, primarily for the more formalised, one-to-one interviews with non-English speakers. Their comprehension of the issues at stake and professional, ethical grounding proved invaluable to the study, where our drives home were filled with dialogue about the interview, assisting me to develop a closer idea of how our individual assumptions and beliefs had coloured our impressions.

The bulk of the study was therefore undertaken alone and involved an immersion into the linguistic environment, which improved my language competence considerably under the tutelage of participants. Translations with patients were still required at times of course, however these were often spontaneously provided by other participants who might also be translating the general meaning to others. This did not always work: once I appealed to a patient standing by and apparently listening to the monologue of one particular person, asking 'what is she saying?'. To which the unconcerned but affable reply was, 'I also do not understand, never mind'. Generally, however, I did understand much of what was being said, the gist was usually caught without too many problems, words falling into specific meaning at a later date, although sometimes irascible Maya, a long-stay patient, would crossly tell me I was *bodoh* (stupid) for not understanding her.

Due to my slow and hesitant use of language I was heavily reliant on the circumstances in which utterances and gestures took place and who responded to speakers or who ignored them (Fabian, 1996). It was some time later that I came across Unni Wikan's (1993) comments on her own very similar position, whereby she utilises a postmodernist debate about whether language is able to fully represent and express the relationship between the self and the external world. Wikan dismisses an ethnographic preoccupation with words, such as is the basis of discourse analysis and argues for a more 'empathic' attitude, commenting that it may instead be necessary to

> Transcend the words, we need to attend to the speaker's intention, and the social position they emanate from, to judge correctly what they are doing (Wikan, 1993: 193).

Empathy combined with good listening and observation skills were put to good use in this study, where the context of communication in relation to the literal message conveyed vital meaning. I came to note, for example, how little substance and attention were granted to patients' words by staff and fellow patients. By contrast the statements of staff were weighty and authoritative, as Robert Desjarlais (1996) notes of desk staff at a shelter for the mentally ill in Boston, USA in his ethnographic study. At Tranquillity, English was used by staff largely as *the* language of medical authority and nearly all nursing staff spoke a formalised English to the ward doctors, but among themselves returned to the locally flavoured English garnished with Malay (Spradley, 1979). Finally, while physical distance was the norm between the medical staff, physical proximity and touch was also used as another dominant and most eloquent medium of communication by many of the women patients. I experienced having my hand held, embraces, pats and strokes and at the other extreme threatened slaps or spitting conveyed a wealth of meaning, which often made verbal communication redundant.

Ethics and fieldwork

Ethical considerations permeated the fieldwork experience, one of the main ones being how far I should involve myself in those events taking place around me which I interpreted as being of a dubious nature. On some occasions, I felt that I should intervene, whilst on others I remained uncertain and kept silent, inducing anxieties about tacit collusion, which remained unresolved. Two short examples serve to illustrate this dilemma quite well. The first took place during an informal chat with a medical assistant who was talking about his job in an animated fashion. Close by a male patient was aiming vicious kicks and blows at another who was cowering without retaliation. It is very likely that this would have continued if I had not quite quickly drawn the medical assistant's attention to what was taking place a few yards behind him. My interference at this point I felt to be perfectly proper behaviour, however on another occasion during the early days of fieldwork I witnessed a woman patient approach a nurse to ask for a sanitary towel. A brief wrestling match ensued while the nurse attempted to expose the woman's naked genitals in public to verify that the patient's menses had really begun. Judging from the patient's reaction this was clearly a humiliating violation of personal privacy, but one in which I did not intervene but instead carefully noted.

The first example shows me in a paternalistic light as the two men were patients who also suffered from learning disabilities. I also assumed at the time that the medical assistant seemed to be momentarily neglecting his duties, perhaps because I was distracting him, and that therefore this accidental omission gave me license to interfere. In the latter case, the emancipatory aims of this study notwithstanding, I was uncertain of how much authority I could bring to bear on the situation, and whether my primary role was to observe or to intervene. Whilst naturally the self-interested thought flickered through my mind that interference between a nurse and her patient would also jeopardise my tenuous standing on the ward, and consequently my study.

Subsequently I witnessed other episodes involving staff and patients that worried me, but more often, I was presented with low-key dilemmas; for example, one woman that I got to know quite well asked me to intercede with the staff on her behalf. Once or twice I did bring these kinds of matters to the attention of the staff, but most of the time I tried to encourage patients to voice their own concerns to the appropriate authority. I wanted to avoid being seen as either an unorthodox member of staff or alternatively as an adopted advocate on patient issues. Thereby I found myself neatly caught in quandaries and dilemmas as a researcher faced with actual instances of oppression in the field. I reasoned that either situation would probably interfere with developing relations with groups of informants, as well as probably contravene my agreed role. Therefore, caught on the horns of a dilemma I also attempted to confine my role to simple observation and did not interfere with events taking place around me, yet the issue remained, perplexing, distressing and irresolvable.

In relation to these kinds of issues, Nettle (1996) describes how she was able to draw clear boundaries between her brief as a researcher and deeper involvement in the concerns of psychiatric patients. While Kleinman (1991) points out the difficulties of managing negative emotions towards events and participants in the field, and that these feelings express personal values through which a process of deeper reflection and analysis is usually distanced by time and place. Kim Lützén, (1996: 79), however, acknowledges that 'holding values in suspension' can be morally ambiguous during times when we should intervene; such situations remain problematic for researchers in terms of ethics and methodology.

Given that research does not inhabit a moral vacuum and weighing up the contingent status of research, my response to this kind of dilemma was clearly a pragmatic one. In order to initiate any level of change I usually resorted to questioning staff about the rationale for policies and practices.

This served a dual purpose of firstly attempting to avoid prejudging behaviours without understanding the context in which they took place. Secondly, I hoped through these means that my questions would spark a process of reflection in my respondent that would challenge established attitudes on the ward leading to change at this point in the hierarchy of power.

The following chapter moves away from the interpersonal negotiations, practical and ethical dilemmas and the basic mechanics of contemporary data gathering to offer a critical review of the nature of asylum care historically, in an attempt to delineate more clearly the connection between eras and philosophies of care, as they relate to the Malaysia.

3
Psychiatry and the colonial enterprise in historical Malaya and Borneo

The historical context in Europe

Specifically aimed psychiatric treatment of mentally ill patients in the West has only been in existence since the Enlightenment, and this type of care has in many ways changed almost out of recognition from early concepts of mental illness and appropriate methods of management. In England prior to the era of the county asylum in the nineteenth century, mental illness was primarily managed at home, the poorhouse, prison or the punitive atmosphere of the workhouse. Scull (1979) argues that, by the mid-eighteenth century, the status of madness was being redefined as a condition subject to medicalised expertise rather than one of individual inadequacy.

This period saw the beginnings of a consciousness that the insane could be treated rather than merely contained. General institutional care in Europe prior to this has been condemned for its brutality, with the mad treated like wild animals, that were moreover judged to be impervious to pain, cold, hunger and foul accommodation.

> The whole system of treatment was also predicated on the assumption that mental patients are habitually disordered, malicious, base creatures. Every attempt was made to force them to renounce their foolishness and bring them to submission by abusing and punishing them (Kraepelin, 1962: 24).

Porter (2006) points out how little research has been done on the care of the insane prior to the eighteenth century. Thus our knowledge of this area remains patchy. Yet the later, and often callous, incarceration of incorrigibles - typified by the frightful descriptions of one James Norris, a 'lunatic' kept for well over a decade encased in leather and metal restraints - saw the concept of the asylum evolve to one in which the asylum in *itself* could be seen as therapeutic and a means of achieving a cure (Scull, 1993). This revolutionary idea followed from the logic of the period, whereby rationality was seen to sweep away the superstitions and rigid social structures of the Middle Ages, articulated, for example, through the measured reasoning of William Battie, a founding member of one of the new public sector asylums, St Luke's Hospital in London (Shorter, 1997).

> Madness is ... as manageable as many other distempers, which are equally dreadful and obstinate, and yet are not looked upon as incurable; such unhappy objects ought by no means to be abandoned, much less shut up in loathsome prisons as criminals or nuisances to the society (Shorter, 1997: 10).

The idea of the 'therapeutic benefits' of the asylum was one that was consequently transported to the American colonies, and in due course to all other corners of the British Empire, including Malaya, over the following two centuries.

Foucault, as is well known, argued that the eighteenth century was the period that saw the establishment of the great and universal 'complicity between government and Church' in Europe, replacing earlier measures of support or oppression of the poor and infirm (Littlewood and Lipsedge, 1989: 32; Foucault, 1966; Foucault, 1976a). In evidence of this Foucault (1966) points to bureaucratically centralised France, where by 1798 there were in existence 177 State sector custodial institutions, of which the most famous were Bicêtre, for male patients, and Salpêtrière for females.

This argument, however, is contested by both Andrew Scull (1993) and Peter Barham (1992) as being unrepresentative of the situation in England at that time, where institutions were largely private, entrepreneurial ventures, rather than State-governed. In accord Shorter (1997) states that there was slow development of the public-sector traditional asylum in England, which numbered only seven charity-run institutions apart from Bethlem and the numerous privately-run institutions. These served to modestly supplement the numerous privately run institutions, where the early version of the 'alienist' practiced or attended the afflicted wealthy in their own home. Furthermore, despite the rise of asylums in England at this time, admission numbers remained remarkably low:

> By 1826, when national statistics became available in England, only minimal numbers of individuals found themselves in either private or public asylums. Not quite five thousand insane people confined in any form, 64 percent of them in the private sector, 36 percent in the public. Bethlem and St Luke's together numbered only 500 patients, and a further 53 insane individuals were in jails – this in a country of 10 million people (Shorter, 1997: 5).

In keeping with the new spirit of optimism towards the asylum as curative, as opposed to segregatory and punitive, the view that insanity could be retrained into rationality manifested itself in a form of care known as 'moral treatment', as exemplified by William Tuke's institution for mentally ill Quakers, 'The Retreat', at York in 1729. Here the emphasis lay equally upon firmness but kindness in dealing with the antics of the insane, helping them to conform to the boundaries of rational behaviour and civil discourse, with work playing an important part in occupying hands and minds (Black, 1988). As Porter (1983: 36) elegantly states, the Enlightenment drew upon the analogies of wider State politics and the individual psyche to create the representation of the 'rational government of the parts, madness the appetites' insurrection'. Foucault's (1971) analysis of power and madness accordingly argues that Tuke's demand for rational behaviour among residents was the less than benign substitution of the (terrifying) freedom of madness from normal constraints by the madman, to the imposition of the crushing awareness of self-responsibility.

Moral treatment was not applied to the mentally ill alone, for in the American colonies it was also considered appropriate care for physical illnesses, in which there was displayed as considerable a concern for moral and spiritual aspects, as for physical rehabilitation (Luchins, 1989).

The ideology behind hospital admissions during this period was consequently based more on 'social and moral criteria than on the nature of the person's illness' (Luchins, 1989: 587). Perhaps not surprisingly, given such rationale, we learn that hospitals in the late eighteenth and early nineteenth century were regarded as highly stigmatising charitable institutions. Moral treatment in hospitals, similar to asylum care under the same philosophy, emphasised the removal of afflicted individuals from the contaminating influences of their home and peer environment, thus rehabilitating them into 'humane, civil, productive and responsible citizens' able to withstand the 'temptations of their neighborhoods' (Luchins, 1989: 587).

The concept of the *ideal* asylum evolved from the eighteenth up to the twentieth centuries and was seen to be one that was designated into functional areas, which in turn would be replicated through reinterpretation in the colonies These areas provided, in literally concrete terms, a means for guiding the patient into the orderly rhythms of normality. The building in itself was seen as a material method of rehabilitation; suitable architecture therefore providing metaphorically the rational parameters necessary for the promotion of rational living (Saris, 1996; Turner, 1992). Lindsay Prior (1993) notes that documentation from as late as the 1940s describes the ideal hospital environment as a completely segregated, self-contained community located in a large, secluded rural area where all categories of patients could be cared for. This may have seemed something of an ideological departure in respect of one of the earliest institutions for the insane - Bethlem (Bedlam) - which as the conurbation grew, would later be more centrally situated in London at Bishopsgate (Ng and Chee, 2006). In the sixteenth century, however, the institution stood slightly beyond the parameters of the compact city.

These enclosed institutions in pastoral settings, to which Prior (1993) refers, historically included not only the mentally ill, but a miscellaneous population comprising the mentally retarded, the sick, vagrants and criminals (Shorter, 1997). The concept of the self-enclosed community offers a chilling description that is immediately recognisable as conforming precisely to Erving Goffman's definition of the 'total institution' (Goffman, 1968: 296; Goffman, 1991).

The humane and rational treatment of the insane could be delivered reasonably well in England and the Empire, with only a limited number of individuals accommodated in asylums. Unfortunately, the early nineteenth century saw a massive rise in admissions – a phenomenon that also occurred in Europe, the American colonies and, as will be seen, at a later date in colonial Malaya as well as in several other colonial psychiatric institutions (Ernst, 2010; Jackson, 2005; Sadowsky, 2003). The late nineteenth-century asylum would of necessity abandon much of the rehabilitative content of care and more importantly would become an increasingly closed community, heavily custodial and characterised by locked wards. Duly these responses to overcrowding would be re-enacted in asylums in the Malayan, Indian subcontinent and African regions (Clark, 1966; Ernst, 2010; Fernando, 2010; Jackson, 2005).

Shorter (1997) states that within the first decade of the nineteenth century there were sixteen new asylums built in the London area alone, including Colney Hatch, which held 2,200 beds and the Hanwell Asylum, West London with 2,600 beds.

> What were intended by early Victorian reformers as small country houses to provide refuge for not much more than one hundred inmates had been transformed by the end of the century into sprawling 'stately homes' that behind their elegant facades reproduced the worst conditions of urban overcrowding (Barham, 1992: xi).

The reason for this enormous increase in the number of detainees in asylums is a highly contested area: for Sutton, asylums in England appear to have been used for a large scale exercise in socio-behavioural control, where they became a 'dumping ground' for the physical and mental wrecks of industrial capitalism (Sutton, 1997: 52). Shorter responds by ascribing the increase to three main factors. Firstly, the enormous rise in neurosyphilis and secondly to a significant increase in alcohol abuse. Finally, Shorter, following Scull, points to a radical change in the structure of the family, which would no longer accommodate the disruptive presence of the insane in its midst (Shorter, 1997; Scull, 1979). Furthermore, Lis and Soly (1996) suggest that upper-class families initiated the search for custodial care for unruly, violent and immoral relatives, followed eventually by proletarian families, and this largely on economic grounds, so that asylum admission would represent only a temporary suspension of labour, particularly in the case of men.

Complicit psychiatry

Historical overviews of the birth of psychiatry have inevitably expanded to include these developments in the colonies; and the transported evolution of asylums from concentrated sites of colonial activity to macro-scale national assimilation and adaptation. Comparisons often depend upon the numbers of psychiatric institutions, trained staff and budget allocation prior to the postcolonial period, with the exponential growth in these areas since, which is constructed as an unqualified good. Accordingly, we learn that while there were only four, albeit very large, psychiatric hospitals in the Dutch East Indies, by the 1970s this number had doubled in Indonesia (Pols, 2006). Likewise, in Pakistan, since Independence the numbers of psychiatric institutions has grown exponentially (Gilani et al., 2005). Deva (2004) in turn reports similar developments that have taken place in Malaysia, of which more will be said.

Goldberg *et al.* (2000) provide a useful context by which to measure these apparent improvements, by pointing out that the overwhelming majority of the world's population live in the developing world and many of these countries have experienced colonialism. Thus, the historiographies of biomedicine have intersected with those of colonial rule; and the latter, as Keller (2001) points out, has been duly strengthened by a Foucauldian analysis of power. Accordingly, the projected mission of British colonialism, for example, that was perceived at the time as fundamentally benevolent and civilising, as well as undeniably profitable, have since been subject to powerful, iconoclastic accusations that have served to sharply refute many of the more benign associations imperialism once boasted of. Thus, the irredeemable evils of empire building have become a guilt-laden, culturally embedded, assumed fact in the contemporary consciousness. Yet such analyses are as captured within a specific socio-historical context, equally as much as that phenomena under study. It is timely to recall then to what extent the greatest admiration, as well as the opprobrium of historians and the informed public, is compelled by sheer fascination when contemplating the mightiest example of administrative, military and cultural hegemony of all: that of the Roman Empire. It is not inconceivable therefore, that emerging revisionist analyses in the 'post' postcolonial future may offer new shades of meaning and alternative interpretations for further consideration in our understanding of colonialism and its influences. Thus, as Keller (2001) advises, the more modest study of colonial psychiatry needs to move beyond over-simplistic accounts of racist oppression by colonials, towards a more nuanced and historically situated analysis in order to do this important topic justice.

A valuable corpus of literature on colonial psychiatry has begun to be consolidated over the past few decades, which provides important insights into formalised psychiatric services offered by the British, French and Dutch colonial authorities across Asia and Africa. Such a wide socio-historical-geographical span inevitably leads to rich, multilayered, diverse and textualised accounts that elicit our critical understanding of the processes, practices and principles underlying the establishment of services and their impact upon local communities. These historiographic studies in turn serve to illuminate ethnographic accounts of psychiatric service users, such as this study, where indigenisation has reshaped service provision to fit a postcolonial landscape, and where the historical thread is less distinct but still visible for tracing back to *a* beginning, if not *the* beginning.

Colonialism has been credited, albeit with much ambivalence, qualification and reservation, with the establishment of modern psychiatric services in its once occupied territories. Pan-Asia and Africa both saw numerous incidents of industry in the introduction of European psychiatry, albeit unevenly and with markedly different standards of care applied across communities. A necessarily brief tour through the literature reveals the extent of this enterprise to bring modern psychiatric care to the indigenous masses.

The imperial machinery, it is argued, was run through the careful coalition of its essential parts, in which psychiatry and medicine in general had a vital role to play in the consolidation of the Empire, along with bureaucratic administration and the militia (Bhugra, 2001).

Accordingly, Roland Littlewood questions how colonial administrations were served by the rising profession of psychiatry developing in parallel in colonised regions.

> We might note, for instance, some affinities between the scientific objectification of illness experienced as disease and the objectification of people as chattel slaves or a colonial manpower, or the topological parallels between the nervous system and imperial order. Both argued for an absence of higher 'function' or sense of personal responsibility among patients and non-Europeans (Littlewood, 2001: 9).

In this analysis colonial authorities viewed subject people as being greatly in need of the new science of psychiatry due to their pathologically morbid tendencies, and generally benighted and ignorant condition. These practices were therefore viewed as an essential part of the armoury that an imperial state could utilise as useful propaganda in aiding the ambitions of notably, although by no means solely, the British Empire.

Dinesh Bhugra (2001) points out that the development of asylums in colonial India were predicated on European notions of medical hierarchy, management and care and governed by enlightened, paternalistic and preferably Anglo-Saxon expertise.

> The ideal psychiatrist, like the ideal colonial officer or plantation owner, was a 'father to his children' (Littlewood and Lipsedge, 1989: 10).

In India we learn that the growth of asylums paralleled historical turmoil, and consequently were built in areas of social unrest with a high colonial presence (Bhugra, 2001). This conflated point is also noted in the more in-depth study by Waltraud Ernst (2010), and is also echoed in accounts of colonial psychiatry from Zimbabwe to Algeria and the Malayan archiepalego. Ernst (2010), however, observes that psychiatric institutions established in the British Raj were primarily there to care for the insane colonial, predominantly army personnel, who had become deranged through a combination of factors, including culture shock, climate differences, homesickness, alcoholism, and the rigours and privations of regular army life overseas, where soldiers were beset with very high disease and mortality rates from a battery of potentially fatal diseases.

While noting that asylum care in India was regarded as generally superior to that offered in the 'home' country, Ernst (2010) comments that strict distinctions were observed between colonial patients and their Indian counterparts in terms of comfort, where in case of Indians overcrowding and squalor were rife. However, equally she notes the prevalent asylum policy of this period, extended to Indian inmates, that maltreatment of patients by staff was strictly forbidden, in accordance with the principles of moral therapy. Ernst (2010), however, argues that the overwhelming scale of the local population caused the insane but innocuous 'native' to be relegated to a life of highly uncertain provision beyond the walls of the asylum. By contrast, those among the colonial insane who did not recover their wits within a certain timespan were regularly repatriated back to the custodial care of asylums in England.

McCulloch (2001) in turn notes the increase in asylums in the European context and the corresponding growth of patient populations in relation to an analysis of the social control of the working classes. He argues, however, that this has little relevance to the development of the asylum system in the colonies where other issues tended to predominate. Furthermore, McCulloch (2001), accused by Keller (2001: 319) of being an 'apologist' for colonialism, goes on to observe that in contrast, the building of asylums in the outback regions of colonial Africa symbolised a wish to emulate the 'civic virtues' of distant metropoles as well as expressing a need to control expatriate and indigenous deviancy (McCulloch, 2001: 79).

Lynette Jackson's (2005) account of Ingutsheni Central Hospital, founded as an asylum in the first decade of the twentieth century in former Southern Rhodesia, offers a graphic analysis of racism in some of the harsh distinctions between the care of white and black patients, particularly in terms of certain forms of treatment, in the period leading up to Independence. Her thesis draws on Franz Fanon's analysis in pointing towards the trauma of colonisation as providing the seeds of psychic disturbance in local populations, where contact with the colonial world could induce insanity in Africans (Jackson, 2005). This in turn chimes with McCulloch's view, according to Keller (2001) that the social transition from traditional, indigenous rural economies to colonised, urban spaces generated psychological trauma in the African population. Curiously, Sadowsky (2003: 212) traces back the origins of such viewpoints to, for example, the 'notorious' J.C. Carruthers who wrote in the 1950s on the psychic impact of encounters with modernity by local Africans. It is indeed an intriguing peculiarity that such similar arguments have been employed diachronically to both castigate, as well as to justify certain colonial psychiatric perspectives of diagnosed mental health problems in indigenous populations.

Notably, Ernst (2010), Bhugra (2001), McCulloch (2001) and Jackson (2005) find that psychiatric admission of the local population was primarily focused on socially troublesome individuals, rather than the harmlessly insane in both colonial India an Africa. The inference is clearly suggestive of a Foucauldian analysis of the exercise of a power against indigenous grass-roots subversion by a threatened imperial State. However, as Keller (2001) in reference to Ernst (2010) points out, the few numbers of patients detained overall, hardly constitutes an effective custodial curb to social subversion. In this vein, Sadowsky in deconstructing this Foucault-inspired conspiratorial aspect of colonialism, adds the observation:

> Although Africans were rarely institutionalized because British officials believed someone to be insane for opposing colonialism, anticolonial sentiments were often taken to confirm that a person already deemed to be acting oddly was, indeed, insane (as already suspected) (Sadowsky, 2003 :213).

Sadowsky goes on to offer an additional critique (2003), arguing that the 'gung-ho' colonial confidence towards the introduction of the clearly beneficial trappings of 'civilisation', such as roads and railways, were expressed with less assurance when it came to mental health provision in the overtly unfamiliar cultural context that colonial Africa represented.

Khanna (2003) draws our attention to the wave of sympathetic protest by French intellectuals, like the existentialist, John Paul Satre, towards France's often brutal colonisation of Algeria, fuelled in part by the compelling critiques of Fanon. While not denying the existence of probable mental illness in his Algerian patients, Fanon argued that effective treatment for colonised patients were negated when administered by the representatives of the enforcing colonial power. Thus, Fanon articulated the interrelationship between colonialism and madness, likening alienation from one's cultural roots, to alienation from one's self (Vaughan, 2007). In discussing Fanon's 'searing indictment of psychiatry' Keller (2007: 4) notes that diagnosed dysfunction by colonial psychiatrists, both British and French, conspicuously failed to contextualise these in relation to macro oppression. Consequently, a more sophisticated analysis is required to understand colonial psychiatry as both a tool of oppression, and as something that could be beneficial, and even conceivably the means of developing emancipatory mechanisms in the geo-political and cultural context (Keller, 2001).

In contrast to these accounts of oppression by invading imperial powers, the convoluted development of mental health treatment in mainland China offers some extraordinary and disturbing insights. In an interesting account by Kam-Shing Yip (2005) we learn that early psychiatric institutions in the late nineteenth century were established by missionaries, firstly in the Guangzhou area. These early initiatives grew, culminating in formal psychiatric training at the Peking Union Medical College in 1932. However, with the demise of the old dynastic order, and the rise of the new People's Republic of China (PRC) in 1949, a root-and-branch revolution of mental health services saw the complete rejection of Westernised 'capitalist' psychiatry. In its stead a more radical *authenticised[1]*, rather than indigenised, 'collective action' was imposed to combat mental illness, now reinterpreted as an individualistic and deviant alienation from established political ideology. Mental health treatment would involve the re-education of the abnormal individual through laceratingly humiliating and excoriating personal criticism by fellow patients and workmates as treatment led by a class-brother/sister psychiatrist with the correct political credentials (Yip, 2005: 108-9).

Kleinman and Kleinman (1999; 1995; Kleinman, 1995) have produced some powerfully compelling accounts of the embodied, psychosocial trauma wrought by the ordeals of Cultural Revolution on individuals since disabled by visceral, unresolved and somatised distress. Collective societal resolution of the more agonising aspects of the Revolution appears to be evaded by a complicit societal amnesia, despite the otherwise complete social transformation of China towards heavy urbanisation and capitalist entrepreneurialism. Today authenticised, culturally grounded therapies like traditional Chinese medicine and Tai Chi co-exist more easily with 'Western' biomedical pharmacology, but psychotherapeutic interventions remain marginalised, despite their apparent utility to alleviate some symptoms of trauma (Yip, 2005).

Colonial psychiatry and anthropology

Sashidharan and Francis (1993) note that the eighteenth century Enlightenment saw not only the development of the new profession of psychiatry but also of theories about race and morbidity. These informed early views of psychiatry and continue, so it is argued, to preoccupy the profession today. The authors assert that while theories of race were traditionally divided into hierarchical relationships, wherein European superiority was contrasted with the inferior, colonised races, these were now recast as theories of deviance revolving around the descendants of former colonised subjects (Sashidharan and Francis, 1993).

In relation to difference and diversity, European observers have long entertained an anthropological interest in regional phenomena and their effects on local Third-World populations. Sadowsky (2003), however, identifies that anthropology as a discipline is itself a product of colonial encounters with new cultures; and that arising from these the concept of cultural relativism has developed.

Cleary and Eaton (1992) and Ong (1995) argue that in Borneo and Malaya anthropology served to aid the efforts of the colonialists in enforcing social control through the categorisation of races. In Sarawak, this led to the eventual segregation of ethnic groups (Cleary and Eaton, 1992). Racial categorisation was also a feature of mainland Malaya under colonial rule; however, the sinister overtone of a eugenics-style agenda at play is questionable. The colonial objectives, articulated in the negotiations for Independence, were to afford 'inalienable genealogical and geographical right to the land and its fruits to the *bumiputera*' to protect their interest from the entrepreunial successes of the tenacious migrants from China and the Indian subcontinent, for example (Baba *et al.*, 2010; Chua, 2007: 271). Despite the ironies of such migration having been encouraged by the colonial authorities in the first place, in order to assist in the development of the economic infrastructure, and to more effectively exploit the resources of the Malayan archipelago, these protective policies were summarily adopted by the new postcolonial government.

The fruitful alliance between anthropology and psychiatry continues, as evidenced, for example, by the renowned work of psychiatrist anthropologist Arthur Kleinman. Emile Kraepelin, for instance, carried out extensive travels in Java and Malaya, noting regional manifestations of mental disorder (McCulloch, 2001). In Sarawak by the mid-twentieth century the position of the 'Government specialist alienist' and director of the Sarawak Mental Hospital was filled by Dr. K.E. Schmidt who brought with him from Europe many of the experimental advances in psychiatric therapies prevalent in that period. In addition, throughout most of his career in the region, Schmidt, infected, it would seem, with the true zeal of the stereotypical colonial psychiatrist, was busily engaged in the study of the ethnic and cultural peculiarities amongst patient populations and published widely on that topic (Chiu *et al.*, 1972; Nissom and Schmidt, 1961; Schmidt, 1964; Schmidt, 1967).

In addition, the psychoanalytic tradition drew inspiration from the colonial enterprise where a bi-directional influence of psychological interpretations can be detected. Although Khanna (2003) rightly insists on parochialising the psychoanalytic tradition as located within a specific historical-cultural moment, the penetrating and appropriating objective of colonialism offered, appropriately, a rich source of symbolic terrain to probe. The alien and unknowable quality of Africa was symbolically used by Freud in describing women's strange sexuality as the 'dark continent' in reference to phraseology by the nineteenth century explorer, Henry Morton Stanley (Khanna, 2003: 49). Psychoanalysis was typically preoccupied with the irrational fixations and neuroses of the immature mind, those of children and potentially women and primitive people as well (Khanna, 2003). Transported from Europe, psychoanalysis rooted tentatively in India and there evolved to reproduce a new indigenised interpretation of Freudian analysis, such as in relation to the Oedipal Complex, where it is the father, rather than the son that is castrated; allowing Keller (2001: 303) to make a pointed political commentary on the patriarchy of the British Raj and attitudes towards it. Pathological conditions exerted a fascination for Europeans abroad, but where madness, unlike in Europe, does not appear to have been viewed as a particularly feminised condition, especially if based on the numbers of admitted women to asylum across ethnic boundaries. Accordingly, Laura Stoler, in reference to Edward Said's analysis of *Orientalism*, indicates that Asian women preoccupied the fantasies of 'the imperial voyeur' in a different context from that which tended to animate the amateur anthropologist of this period (Stoler, 1991: 54). However, as Keller (2001) elucidates, Ernst (2010) explains this anomaly as the constructed notion of the symbolic feminisation of the subject nation yielding inevitably to the masculine authority of the imperial powers. (2010). Instead, the conditions of indigenous women in relation to mental disorders were subsumed under those of generic male conditions, with rare exceptions, such as that shown towards the phenomenon of *latah* in the Malayan regions, defined as a nervous affliction characterised by involuntary verbal and bodily repetitions, frequently obscene in nature (Winzeler, 1995).

Latah, in its passive, imitative, non-voluntary and mechanical manifestations, was seen primarily as a disorder of Malay and eventually Dayak women (Spores, 1988; Winzeler, 1995). Ronald Simons (1996) by contrast, argues that *latah* is not a condition confined to a specific culture or region solely, but is far from being unknown as a startle response in the West as well. Culture merely dictates the form and degree of the reaction, as well as conferring whatever benefits (or otherwise) may be conferred upon the 'sufferer'. If correspondingly downplayed in the West, *latah* appears to have a distinct social role to play in Southeast Asia (Simons, 1996). In this vein, Aihwa Ong (1990) describes how *latah*, once traditionally associated with older Malay women, has become a common feature amongst young

Malay, female industrial workers caught between conflicting, cultural gender norms. Here *latah* appears to act both as a generalised indicator of tension as well as a possibly that of resistance to these political and cultural contradictions.

Colonial enthusiasts, both contemporary and historical, have long expressed curiosity about such local phenomena as *koro*: an hysterical anxiety that the sufferer's genitals or nipples are fatally receding, and the phenomenon of *amok* as well. These were being increasingly viewed as simply bizarre local manifestations of known European disorders, albeit demonstrated at a more basic, primitive level (Littlewood, 2001; Mo et al., 1995); although one serious outbreak of *koro* in Singapore was noted as late as 1967 (Ng and Chee, 2006). Winzeler (1995) goes on to argue that this perceived tenuous commonality with Europeans and their mental disorders would not suspend European value judgements concerning Malayan people and their propensities towards mental illness.

> In Malayanist versions of Orientalism, sensuality and femininity ... were seldom raised, but instability was given great emphasis. It was axiomatic that Malays, Javanese and other Malayan peoples were by nature 'sensitive to the slightest insult,' 'volatile,' preoccupied with maintaining balance and composure and so forth. Such psychological tendencies were held to be in part a matter of inherent character and in part a consequence of despotic political rule and a rigidly hierarchical social order that was to be changed through the creation of a new way of life under European guidance (Winzeler, 1995: 4).

In this analysis, therefore, colonial rule could be seen as imposing a fundamentally civilising and benevolent power on territorial possessions that would sweep away regional and traditional tyranny, and bring order and medical help to local populations, a view which Ernst (2010) dismisses as mere mythology. The issue of *amok* demonstrates this point in its description, as attributed to an English physician in 1891, as being a 'blind furious homicidal mania' that was 'peculiar to the Malay race' (J Teoh, 1971: 20).

Amok was considered not only a disorder of the Malay (as well as the Javanese) individual but one that was peculiar to men and dishonoured men at that.

> When the Malay feels that a slight or insult has been put upon him ... He broods over his trouble, till, in a fit of madness, he suddenly seizes a weapon and strikes out blindly at everyone he sees - man, woman or child, often beginning with his own family (Swettenham, 1906: 143).

Murphy states, however, that incidents of amok increased in parallel with the colonisation of settlements by Europeans in the eighteenth and early nineteenth century (1973). Although in rural areas amok was still considered an honourable response to intolerable triggers, in the Europeanised urban areas, the social factors were ignored in favour of explanations pointing towards insanity or perhaps somatised physiological conditions. By the 1930s a general diagnosis of schizophrenia was applied to the condition, which by this time had become comparatively rare (Murphy, 1973). The marked decline of cases of *amok*, standing in comparison with its former and rising prevalence, conforms with Golberg's observation that the medicalisation of madness could usefully be employed to support State policy, in this case that of colonialism (Goldberg, 1999).

Western responses to *amok* were divided, with opinions varying between whether this sort of indiscriminate slaughter could be classified as plain crime or insanity; medical opinion eventually veering towards the latter (Hatta, 1996; Spores, 1988). Commensurate with Murphy and Winzeler's arguments, for Spores the gradual demise of *amok* was related to the enormous social changes taking place in feudal Malaya through the imposition of colonial law and order. This, combined with the medicalisation of *amok*, resulted in colonial authorities branding the *amok* runner a lunatic rather than a notorious anti-hero, with all the associated stigma that this conjured up for Europeans and imparted to colonial subjects (McCulloch, 2001).

The colonial psychiatrist therefore found himself in the powerful position of becoming the undisputed 'arbiter of deviance', redefining behaviours previously thought of as little more than local oddities towards classifications of mental disorders, from mild neuroses and hysterias, to the seriously deviant and criminally insane (Romanucci-Ross, 1997a: 18).

> Psychiatry, with its function of defining, maintaining and 'treating' psychological disorder, often identified in the context of social disorder, provides the scientific basis and the legislative and therapeutic justification for a particular approach in dealing with madness. Furthermore, by asserting its expertise in dealing with madness, psychology provides the glue that binds the individually deviant behaviour in the socially sanctioned procedures for incarceration (Sashidharan and Francis, 1993: 98).

Psychiatric opinions could therefore be seen as a useful tool, one that aided and empowered colonial authorities to apply methods of control towards labelled deviant individuals on the grounds of civil order.

The anthropological and medical curiosity towards regional behaviours reframed as 'mental disorders' have continued to excite psychiatric interest for Western and Western-trained psychiatrists. In the mid to late twentieth century interest in the so-called 'cultural-bound syndromes' generated large-scale research intent on establishing classifications that were strongly reminiscent of the endeavours of colonial psychiatry:

> The extent to which such patterns could be fitted into a universal schema depended on how far the medical observer was prepared to stretch a known psychiatric category (Littlewood, 2001: 4).

Consequently, the interest in culture-bound syndromes can be read as providing continuing examples of perceived 'otherness' for Western observers, which become dislocated from the meaning associated with their manifestations. Culture-bound syndromes are viewed as strange exotica and reinterpreted within a framework of classification to make them more intelligible to unfamiliar audiences. According to Naomi Selig (1988: 96) the spate of cross-cultural psychiatric studies looking at the incidence of schizophrenia globally in the 1960s continued to exemplify the modern day 'colonial stance'.

The attempt to identify universals in mental illness formed the basis of the World Health Organization (WHO) International Pilot Study of Schizophrenia in 1966. A significant finding to come out of this report was that, contrary to expectations, diagnosed schizophrenics in some developing countries had a better prognosis of recovery than those in the developed countries of the West. A follow-up study two years later supported this finding (Sartorius *et al.*, 1977). Other psychiatric studies in cross-cultural variables have specifically attempted to focus on the connection between psychiatric disorders and the 'sociocultural' environment using very large statistical samples of 'different groups of people' (Leighton and Murphy, 1966: 3). Both the WHO report of 1966 and cross-cultural psychiatry have been subjected to sharp criticisms, largely on methodological grounds. Kleinman (1988: 14-15) points out how disease has been schematised into professional taxonomies, which when applied cross-culturally have fallen methodologically foul of what he describes as the 'category fallacy': that of applying cultural specific diagnostic nosologies onto culturally diverse samples. This unwarranted application of nosologies persistently ignores the underlying point that *biomedicine* itself is merely another form of ethno-medicine but is nonetheless 'treated as a universal construct' (Nichler, 1992: xii; Crandon-Malamud, 1997). This underlying assumption is clearly conveyed by descriptions of cross-cultural psychiatry:

As an underlying principle [my italics] we take an attitude of inclusiveness in these regards just as we do in dealing with the range of psychiatric phenomena as defined by Western thought...it seems unnecessary to waver in the face of cultural relativism as though we completely lacked valid standards of functioning' (Leighton and Murphy, 1966:12-13).

Dawn Terrell (1994) consequently highlights the basic assumption of the study: that there is a universal identification of abnormality, this provides both the baseline for the study, and effectively begs the question by so doing.

In connection with these points and in reference to contemporary Black dissent regarding psychiatric practices and assumptions in the West, Chakraborty argues that for the most part modern psychiatry has failed to grasp the implications of ethnicity, and continues to interpret cultures from a Western ethnocentric viewpoint only.

For most psychiatrists culture has meant odd happenings in distant places that did not apply to them. The difference that they found in other cultures was ascribed to childlike behaviour, magical thinking, or inferior social or psychological development. Old healing traditions were thought to be unscientific; healers were judged to be abnormal or psychotic; and handbooks were written on how to study psychiatric symptoms among 'natives' (Chakraborty, 1991: 12).

Fernando *et al.* (1998) argue that contemporary as well as historical psychiatry continues to be a powerful instrument of social control of perceived and labelled deviants in society and go on to take issue with the racial bias that is built into psychiatric diagnosis. This, the authors contend, adopts stereotypic assumptions concerning the inherent alien nature, inferiority and dangerousness of black people leading to custodial care (Fernando *et al.*, 2005). In this way racist assumptions from the past inform the present and duly resonate with Littlewood and Lipsedge's point that the primitive being is already 'in a sense ill', or in other words, infantile and maladjusted and therefore less prone to mental illness (Littlewood and Lipsedge, 1989: 34). Accordingly, Kleinman (1988: 37) recounts that depression has been seen by 'paternalistic and racialist' psychiatrists as uncommon in India and Africa due, we are led to infer, to assumptions concerning the primitive and non-introspective cast of mind of non-Westerners (Fernando, 1995). Such views tally with the observation of Dr Schmidt in describing 'Land Dayaks' (the Bidayuh) as fundamentally superstitious, fearful and 'ignorant' (Schmidt, 1964: 142; Schmidt, 1967: 357).

The racist overtones of such views are transparently obvious to modern-day scholars, but the cultural presumptions inherent in contemporary generic biomedicine, embodied in every-day medical practice and malpractice with minority groups, are being increasingly testified to in medical journals (Bhugra, 1997; Bose, 1997; Cohen, 1999; McLaughlin and Braun, 1998; Murphy, 1978; Vanchieri, 1998).

Furthermore, through historical associations and contemporary training, the racism of ethnocentricity is not confined to the West but is duly exported to other countries. Acharyya, for instance, identifies psychiatric care with modern-day colonialism: whereby 'Third-World psychiatrists' trained in Britain incorporate the dominant paradigm so completely that they find difficulties in evolving new methods of dealing with mental illness within their own culture (Acharyya, 1996: 339). Contemporary critiques of racist assumptions and values in psychiatry form a useful prism to view modern-day practices in both the West and in former colonies such as Malaysia.

Madness and gender in multicultural Malaya

The rise of the modern psychiatric movement in Malaysia derives its origins from its colonial heritage. Britain, as well as the Dutch in what is now Indonesian Borneo (Kalimantan), were busily exporting European concepts of illness and contemporary methods of care to their colonies. It should be noted from the outset that, as discussed in Chapter One, the developments in colonial Malaya were not greatly influential in East Malaysia. The position of Sarawak under the Brooke rule, for instance, can be seen to be an historical anomaly that was not specifically connected to British imperialism in Malaya, but that at the time the settlement of Singapore was counted as part of Crown territories in the Malayan region. The accession of Sarawak to the new Federation of Malaysia in 1963 tied its future firmly to that of the Peninsula, and eventually Singapore claimed independence from the Federation of Malaysia. All this lay in the future however, and prior to this period Sarawak evolved at a quite different pace, and under a very different system, in which the development of psychiatry appears to have played a very minor role in comparison to colonial Malaya.

European health care in Malaya was first introduced into urban areas and only progressed to remote rural locations with the expansion of colonial authority (Manderson, 1996). This is in keeping with general colonial policy that health care should primarily serve the expatriate population, whether civilian or military; and in this respect care of insanity was treated in the same spirit, with the siting of asylums in areas of British influence (Bhugra, 2001; McCulloch, 2001). Consequently, the first recorded lunatic asylum in Malaya was built near the regimental hospital under the auspices of the colonial authorities in Penang, a Crown possession for some decades since 1786, to cater, it is claimed, for primarily syphilitic European sailors (Baba, 1992; Deva, 1992). By 1829 however, there were a mere 25 inmates in the Penang asylum, 23 men and two women, almost all being Chinese and Indian (Tan and Wagner, 1971).

Commensurate with the rapid expansion of the asylum system earlier in nineteenth-century England, the rapidly growing colonial settlement of Singapore saw the sequential building of several asylums, commencing with a comparatively small 'Insane Hospital' in 1841, where previously the insane were abandoned to the indifferent care of the local gaol (Ng and Chee, 2006, Tan and Wagner, 1971; Shorter, 1997). Eventually this situation culminated in the establishment of the large 'New Mental Hospital' in 1928 (Ng and Chee, 2006). However, in the nineteenth and early twentieth century, despite colonial concerns that asylums were required in Singapore, this does not imply that the perceived prevalence of insanity was comparable with that of England in 1900, where it was almost 30% higher than in the Singaporean community (Teoh, 1971).

By 1887, however, an English psychiatrist by the name of William Gilmore Ellis was appointed to take charge of a newly built asylum in the recently established colonial settlement of Singapore (Ng and Chee, 2006). This building, constructed in 1885 on the Sepoy Lines, replaced the original asylum of 1862, which, it seems, had been built to cater for predominantly Asian migrant labour following a murder at the local gaol. Due to overcrowding of the asylum, however, apparently a policy of repatriation of chronically ill Chinese and Indian inmates commenced, duly resonating with the accounts of Ernst and Jackson in this regard.

A further institution was opened in Penang in 1860 but this did not remain for long, with the Sepoy Lines asylum at Singapore being subsequently obliged to absorb their internee population following closure (Murphy, 1971). The next institution on Peninsular Malaya was not established until circa 1910 when the Central Mental Hospital was built in Tanjong Rambutan, a few miles from the tin-mining town of Ipoh in Perak (Tan and Wagner, 1971). Its name was changed to Hospital Bahagia in 1971.

Returning to Gilmore Ellis' Singapore asylum, admissions in the late nineteenth century were noted to come from as far afield as Bangkok and Australia, where, in the latter case at least, psychiatric services were considered to be far more rudimentary (Teoh, 1971). Although in South Australia, at least, there had been an attempt to model them on British counterparts as a need for asylum care was recognised due to the repercussions of migration on the mental health of colonial settlers (Piddock, 2004). Apart from the Straits Settlements (Penang and Singapore), cases were referred from the States of Johore, Malacca and Selangor; the quality of early psychiatric services in Malaya at this time was evidently by no means deficient in comparison with other nations (Teoh, 1971). Even at the original Singapore asylum the number of psychiatric beds per capita was roughly equivalent to that of Britain and ahead of America, with conditions for patients considerably preferable compared to the community and institutional abuses of the insane in North America (Geller and Harris, 1994; Murphy, 1971). A fact perhaps not so surprising when put in the context of asylums in the British Raj, which were often superior to those in Britain and supported by comparatively enlightened policies and rapid responses to reform (Keller, 2001; Ernst 2010). This, notwithstanding a revisionist critique of the colonial authorities neglect of the vagrant mentally ill Indian beyond the walls of the asylum, and the overcrowding and racially-based differences in treatment within them (Ernst, 2010)

To return to historical Singapore, the types of admission to the new asylum were varied, with the first case of neurosyphilis in the Asian local population noted in 1906. By comparison in England, Shorter (1997) argues that neurosyphilis rose to epidemic proportions swelling the numbers of nineteenth-century asylums and resulting in mania, paralysis, dementia and death, with further cases of morbidity due to a rise in alcohol abuse. Accordingly, from the beginnings of the twentieth century the socio-economics of the period dictated that 20% of all admissions to the Sepoy Lines asylum were suffering from signs of neurosyphilis. Whilst equally by 1906 in grim comparison it was noted that similarly alcoholic psychosis was beginning to replace illnesses caused by opium consumption (Teoh, 1971).

Prior to Gilmore Ellis' supervision of the new Singapore asylum the original hospital in Stamford Raffles' Singapore had an enviable discharge rate of 89% with most cases admitted suffering from acute psychotic attacks after the use of opium and other narcotics; this situation was not to last however (Murphy, 1971). Madness and ethnicity were already viewed by medical authorities of the time as following certain racially determined lines, and consequently Chinese migrant workers were perceived as suffering from their own distinct forms of insanity and increasingly so, as Victor Purcell states:

Insanity among the Chinese was attributed to drinking, opium-smoking and gambling, and in some measure to speculation ... Chinese lunatics suffered from dementia mostly, whereas the other races had mania, the former being due to gambling and opium-smoking (Purcell, 1948: 65).

Gambling, use of opium and more notoriously venereal diseases were a feature of life for nineteenth-century colonial Malaya where migrant labour was overwhelmingly made up of male Asian workers from China and the Indian subcontinent. These men were largely brought to work in tin mines, on estates and railways, and in small private enterprises, although in Sarawak Chinese farming skills were sought (Chew, 1990). By contrast, immigrant women were largely brought to work in brothels serving Asian migrant and white expatriate masculine needs (Manderson, 1996). Prostitution however, carried its own penalties in the form of syphilis, which was initially a rare occurrence amongst non-Europeans.

General Paralysis of the Insane, a syphilitic infection of the brain which causes insanity, was never seen among Asiatics. Practically all cases were among those of European stock and it was then considered that the disease was peculiar to Europeans only and was a disease of civilised life running at high pressure (Teoh, 1971: 20).

The inference here being that the *pressures* that the white expatriate community suffered from were similar to those of the Asian expatriate community, whereby socially sanctioned conjugal relationships were unlikely in a social environment characterised by a lack of eligible females. British civil servants in Malaya, in common with other colonial regions, required permission to marry from their employers and this only after many years of service, which consequently gave rise to the institution of concubinage of local women (Stoler, 1991). This, Stoler argues, was an expedient policy that preserved the health of expatriate males and helped to secure their continued employment and contentment in foreign regions.

In relation to this point, Teoh notes that the majority of admissions to the Singapore asylum at this time were in an appalling state of health; with women admissions, few though they may have been, in the worst physical condition of all (1971). A plausible inference may be drawn under the circumstances that these were due to the ravages of a life of prostitution and its concomitant hazards, as much as from any other form of disease and hardship.

The low admission rates in Singapore at the turn of the nineteenth century have been in part attributed to the low percentage of women admissions, and this in turn due to very few numbers of women per capita in the community at this time, where the first case of puerperal insanity was admitted to the asylum as late as 1888 (Teoh, 1971; Ng and Chee, 2006). This has been estimated as standing in the region of three women to every 10 men, and as such represents a comparable situation to that of other conurbations of British influence in colonial Malaya during this general period (Tan and Wagner, 1971; Teoh, 1971). Nonetheless, this was not an isolated national anomaly, for in colonial Nigeria, there were three times as many male patients in psychiatric care as females, and where originally in the Ingutsheni Lunatic Asylum, no provision had been made for women at all (Sadowsky, 1999, Jackson, 2005).

These therefore, as Keller (2001) observes, create some significantly interesting anomalies when correlated with feminist studies of admission rates of women in England during the era, whereby according to Kromm (1994: 507), it denoted 'a clear shift in the understanding of madness as a gendered disorder'. She goes on to argue that theatrical and pictorial representations increasingly depicted woman as the embodiment of madness in various postures of *melancholia* as opposed to *mania* (Kromm, 1994). Furthermore, Showalter (1985) argues that the over-representation of madness amongst women was far from being merely a nineteenth-century and twentieth-century phenomenon, but existed from the seventeenth century onwards.

To rehearse the analysis of these feminist studies of the feminisation of madness Denise Russell (1995: 18), in support of Kromm's assertion that there existed a preponderance of women in British public mental hospitals in the nineteenth century, considers the late eighteenth-century interest in 'specifically female problems' as an origin of perceiving insanity as a gendered condition. It is argued that these forms of feminine pathology were dominated by the medical preoccupation with female sexuality and moral purity. In turn, this continues as a dominant discourse in relation to the labelling of women as suffering from mental illness (Barnes and Bowl, 2001; Ussher, 1991).

Joan Busfield (1994), however, contests the assertion of overwhelming numbers of nineteenth-century women in asylum care, and instead asserts that at least in relation to that century the empirical evidence pointing to proportional differences between male and female admission data is quite small. Statistical evidence notwithstanding, diagnosed insanity and high admission rates in the asylum system related to gender depended heavily on the institutionalised perception of woman as essentially associated with the likelihood of insanity.

> Yet the Victorian era marked an important change in the discursive regimes that confined and controlled women, because it was in this period that the close association between femininity and pathology became firmly established with the scientific, literary and popular discourse: madness became synonymous with womanhood (Ussher, 1991: 64).

While the debate concerning the precise numbers of women in asylum care in previous centuries will no doubt continue, there has been little dissent concerning the claim that there has been a universal predominance of women diagnosed with mental illness in the twentieth century (Miles, 1988; Ramon, 1996; Ussher, 1991). Phyllis Chesler (1996: 46) baldly states that more women are being hospitalised with a diagnosis of mental illness than 'at any other time in history'. These diagnoses are, she argues, predominantly affective depressive disorders in keeping with women's subdued and passive presence in society, a topic also explored by Redfield Jamison (1996) in her personal account of bipolar depression. Chesler goes on to allude to the continuing dichotomised perceptions that have persisted, lying between the socially accepted, rewarded but inadequate role of the passive, melancholic female and her antithesis: that of the deplored voluble, 'aggressive', masculinised female counterpart.

> When female depression swells to clinical proportions, it unfortunately doesn't function as a role-release or respite. For example ... 'depressed' women are even less verbally 'hostile' and 'aggressive' than non-depressed women; their 'depression' may serve as a way of keeping a deadly faith with their 'feminine' role (Chesler, 1996: 51).

Wetzel (2000) stands in agreement with Jennie Williams (1999) in arguing that in both the developed and developing world, conditions of oppression affect women living in patriarchal societies, such as Malaysia. These forms of oppression towards women include low status, poverty and exploitation, sexual violence and other acts of human rights violation (Barnes and Bowl, 2001; Wetzel, 2000). Other critiques have noted the relationship between mental distress and the oppression that marriage may impose on women, together with the escalated risk factor connected with the role of motherhood (Ramon, 1996; Ussher, 1991). This has accordingly resulted in a global bias towards a high risk of diagnosis of mental illness for women and their subsequent admission to institutional care.

> Long term psychiatric intervention (based upon psychosexual theories) has
> been inappropriately applied to women throughout the world, when their
> real problems were poverty, violence and economics (Wetzel, 2000: 209).

Apart from the issue of gender bias, a further issue of interest for this study lies in the ethnic breakdown of admission rates during this period and subsequent decades. For example, in 1900 the Singapore asylums largely held Chinese and Indian migrants who formed the vast majority of inmates (Teoh, 1971). It is claimed that this situation continued over the next century and was comparable with other asylums in Malaya, such as in Penang (Tan and Wagner, 1971). The implications of continuing bias in this regard is considered in this study, in reference to patient admission at Hospital Tranquillity.

In relation to the issue of ethnic preponderance in contemporary psychiatric care in the West, a relatively small but important body of critique considers the issue of mental illness and the impact of migration and that of cultural dislocation, together with the effects of consequential separation of individuals from their supportive networks. Such analyses focus on the significance of ethnic bias of psychiatry in Britain where British-born men from African-Caribbean background have been predominancely diagnosed with schizophrenia (Nazroo, 1997; Rack, 1982). Furthermore, an interesting aspect of the escalated ethnic presence in psychiatric services noted in Britain, and which appears to hold significant import for modern Malaysia, is that subsequent generations are also at greater risk of diagnosis and hospitalisation, despite a level of familiarisation and acculturation in the adopted alien culture (Barnes and Bowl, 2001). This said, Ramon (1996) highlights the issue of class as being a further factor to consider along with ethnicity and migration. She argues that elements such as education and, presumably, upward social mobility can act as protective factors countering the effects of migration and cultural dislocation (Ramon, 1996). Suman Fernando (1995, 1999), however, draws a general conclusion of institutionalised racism encountering cultural difference; while others have considered the phenomenon in terms of actual illness and social stressors. In this vein Ajita Chakraborty (1991: 1208) condemns the 'value-based and often racist undercurrents in psychiatry' and goes on to note the fundamental tolerance of mental illness amongst families in India, with the inference that stigma is a persistent effect of Western colonial values. This in turn tends to corroborate the psychiatric assumption that most South-Asian psychiatric patients in Britain have a supportive family network and enjoy what Nazroo describes as a 'protective culture', having fewer mental-health needs than other immigrants (Nazroo, 1997: 7). Thus resonating with Teoh's assumption that separation from 'stable and emotional family support' represented a significant risk factor for Indian male migrants in colonial Malaya (Teoh, 1971: 28).

Finally, in contemporary Britain Chinese psychiatric service users have equally been subject to stereotyping, in terms of the assumption that they enjoy a supportive and insular family network, leading to the relative abandonment of carers by the support services (Yee and Shun Au, 1997). In view of the Chinese diaspora and the issue of Chinese asylum admissions in colonial Malaya and Borneo, these latter-day assumptions may contain useful references in understanding the position of Chinese patients in the modern Malaysian psychiatric institution, as represented by Hospital Tranquillity (Kleinman, 1988b).

Back in nineteenth-century Singapore, Gilmore Ellis brought with him contemporary notions of therapeutic care that involved rehabilitative exercises, such as occupational labour; in keeping with British values of the day. These in all likelihood were gender normative activities, and for women revolved around the skills of the good housewife, and which are enacted on hospital wards to this day, as will be discussed further in Chapter Five (Gittins, 1998; Witz, 1992). Gilmore Ellis apparently diverted a considerable amount of Victorian energy and new enthusiasm to improving conditions for the mentally ill commensurate with up-to-date British practices:

> In the first year he abolished strait jackets, got 87% of the patients occupied in one way or another, usually at rope-making or weaving in the workshops, instituted a new and better system of record keeping, prosecuted an attendant for ill treating a patient, and arranged for a Chinese *Wayang* to come and give entertainment (Murphy, 1971: 16).

In Penang, it would seem that such rehabilitative therapies had equally been introduced to patients there. A fascinating insight from a nineteenth century British superintendent who had served at asylums in both Penang and Calcutta stated that the ethnically diverse patients in Penang were far more amenable to 'voluntary manual work' than were the Bengalese patients or their Eurasian counterparts, in his experience (Ernst, 2010: 63).

In nineteenth century Singapore even the rudimentary after-care of discharged patients was not neglected; however, despite all these therapeutic improvements, Gilmore Ellis could not prevent a very high death rate from cholera and beri-beri amongst inmates. Acute cases with a rapid discharge rate were not typical admissions, as had been seen in the earlier Singapore institution. Now psychiatric chronicity and physical morbidity were the main characteristics of patients at the new asylum, a situation that would be replicated in the later running of psychiatric hospitals of colonial Kenya in the 1920s (McCulloch, 2001; Murphy, 1971). The high mortality rate caused by cholera and beri-beri epidemics ravaged the internee population. They were brought under control only to be subsequently replaced by syphilis and tuberculosis, so that the death rate was never below 20% and on occasions rose to 50% of admissions. Gilmore Ellis's response was not complacent, where his own scientific investigations failed, saltwater baths and the curative effects of visits to the seaside succeeded in reducing the mortality rates quite considerably (Murphy, 1971).

In subsequent eras, these fairly benevolent regimes would be overtaken by new forms of treatment such as insulin coma therapy and lobotomy that, as Tai-Kwang Woon dryly notes, 'did not bring any transient hope to the patients or stirred the enthusiasm of the staff' (1971: 31). He goes on to note that medication was used to subdue and control patients, and where this failed, restraints in the form of strait jackets were applied. In the case of Hospital Tranquillity treatment included liberal uses of electro-convulsive therapy (ECT), supplemented by sessions of psychotherapy, under the therapeutic regime of the resident colonial alienist of the period.

Gilmore Ellis's contribution to psychiatric care in Malaya can be seen to have been very much based in the tradition of moral treatment, whereby humane treatment and structured activities were seen to be a highly necessary component in achieving a 'cure'. Unfortunately these early improvements were not sustained and deterioration in care in association with larger admissions began to take place (Teoh, 1971). In the West the loss of the earlier optimism towards effecting a cure for mental illness caused demoralisation amongst pioneering psychiatric professionals by the end of the nineteenth century (Shorter, 1997). This loss of vision could also be seen to be taking its toll on the standards of care even in the new Singapore asylum during this period. By 1909 Ellis had left to take up a new post as Chief Medical Officer in the settlement and a new chapter was opened in psychiatric care in colonial Malaya (Teoh, 1971).

Borneo: Disease, disasters, colonial rule and colonial medicine

Our best accounts of the development of Western medicine *per se* can be found amongst accounts of Dutch imperialism in Borneo; and these are very largely concerned with predominant diseases and their impact on local populations, rather than the more esoteric area of mental disorders, which are referred to solely in passing. This is not to suggest that there existed a dearth of alternative treatment in the region during this period of Dutch imperial expansion. On the contrary, the literature indicates that there was already a wide variety of healing traditions in Borneo and likewise in Malaya (Gullick, 1987; Humholtz, 1991).

Western ethnographic accounts describing shamanistic[2] rituals and the 'derided gullibility' of native audiences in the Borneo region have been in circulation since the nineteenth century (Barrett, 1993: 247). Gullick (1987), however, in writing of the early contact between Malay communities and the colonial powers on the Peninsula in the nineteenth century, comments that for these communities their attitude towards European medical practice tended to be purely pragmatic. This does not imply that the role of the Malay traditional healer, the *bomoh* or *pawing*, was seriously impinged upon - despite Islamic disapproval at a perceived subversion of monotheism through a belief in the teeming existence of spirit beings (*hantus*) (Gullick, 1987). Traditional *adat*, however, ensured the survival of the role, and the *bomoh* was, and continues to be, considered a very useful and skilled individual.

The rich diversity of religious and spiritual traditions in the region continues to fascinate anthropologists; perhaps now even more so, since over time these have been under threat from the encroaching religious hegemonies of Christianity and Islam through conversion and intermarriage (Jehom, 2001). In turn, however, the curative methods of the shaman/spirit medium and priest may be seen to have been challenged by that of biomedicine. As a point of interest, contemporary research continues to confirm that the use of traditional healers amongst the main ethnic groups of Malaysia (and the region in general) is far from being in danger of disappearance (Barrett, 1993; Bentelspacher *et al.*, 1994; Fidler, 1993; Laderman, 1992; 1996; Lewis, 1995; 1997; Wintersteen *et al.*, 1997).

Furthermore, traditional healers, who are frequently greatly respected individuals, can be found practising across ethnic divides. They often continue to be the first recourse for patients, rather than conventional biomedicine, and this holds true for psychological concerns as much as purely physical complaints (Razali, 1995; 1997; Razali *et al.*, 1996).

Anthropologists, psychologists and psychiatrists have long been interested in the enigmatic figure of the shaman. While, Lewis claims that while the mental health specialists have extended their interest into anthropology[3], anthropologists themselves reject explanations that overtly smack of the psychologising of ethnic groups and communities (Lewis, 1995). Such an obdurate attitude by anthropologists may partially be explained by former diagnoses of shamans as neurotic and indeed even psychotic, while their communities have been seen as 'anomic' and 'sick' (Lewis, 1995: 162). Silverman's (1967) well-known description of shamans as 'compensated neurotics' who have experienced and overcome psychological crises successfully, is nonetheless not an altogether unsympathetic interpretation. In this analysis the individual's crisis is transformed into a distinctive, socially useful and respected role through cultural acceptance and incorporation.

The consequence has been that, as Barrett (1993) reports, few anthropologists are willing to ascribe pathological judgements to the people they study. That said, in writing of the Kayans of Central Borneo, Rousseau (1993) comments that shamans who are considered to be the more peculiar by their communities are equally considered the *most* effective. Additionally, Bernstein (1993: 187-188) comments on the 'psychoneurotic' hysterical dramatics of the female Taman shamans of West Kalimantan, concluding that these are based in repressed sexuality. Gender, sexuality and status come to the fore once again, in relation to the psychological stability of these shamans, who, to reiterate, are more likely to be female and of lower status than the comparable but higher-status profession of the priesthood:

> Additionally .... the overall tendency is for priests and priestesses to be 'normal' ... and for shamans ... to be 'abnormal' or troubled at one time or another (Barrett, 1993: xxv).

In further reference to culture and gender norms, Malay *bomohs* are particularly in demand in dealing with the needs of women and children, both of whom are regarded as having lesser *semangat* (variously described as a 'universal spirit' (Laderman and Roseman, 1996: 116) or 'life force' (Peletz, 1995: 92), than those of men, making them more likely to fall prey to spirit possession and illness (Ong, 1990). Lewis (1995), for example, describes how the *bomohs* of Kelantan, West Malaysia, mediate in soothing the stresses caused by the sexual politics between men and women. Female clients fall predominantly into three categories: brides in arranged marriages, the position of first wives in polygamous unions and the situation of divorcees and widows. Laderman and Roseman (1996: 126) in turn describe how the *bomoh's* skills are also used to release the tension caused by 'unsatisfied sexual cravings'. Such powerful appetites as these do not, however, belong to the domain of men, so much as those of women:

> Virtually all women, moreover, hold that women 'need to'- and do in fact – have a stronger sense of 'shame' (*malu*) than men since, if they did not, they would be 'like wild animals' (*macam haiwan*) and chaos would reign throughout the world (Peletz, 1995: 94).

Cure is achieved through the *main peteri*, a Malay séance in which sound, through chants, song and instruments is used as a dominant medium of treatment (Laderman and Roseman, 1996).

The possession of the soul by spirits and the need for restoration by the healer is a an overarching belief across many ethnic groups in the Malayan region, albeit one that is subject to many fine distinctions and diversity of detail. Sacred rituals, however, serve to order the relations between those of men and women within social hierarchies. Of great importance is the demarcation between the worlds of the living and the dead, as a dangerous incursion from the non-living is responsible for illness and disorder. A very frequently performed ritual in Sarawak is that of the *serará bunga*, an Iban mourning ceremony in which flowers are used to achieve this necessary distinction (Barrett, 1993: 240). This ceremony is one that is commonly used in cases of mental illness and many of the patient participants in this study had experienced this form of treatment, regardless of ethnic boundaries.

Despite the continuing popularity of traditional healing rituals they occupy an ambiguous and contradictory position in contemporary Malaysian society. While medical practitioners are usually openly dismissive about the efficacy of traditional cures they are unable and often unwilling to overtly oppose them, and it is not uncommon for medical personnel to seek out such cures for themselves, albeit usually covertly.

Although the supposed gullibility of communities like the Iban is taken issue with, Barrett argues that in fact scepticism of the *manang's* abilities during the performance (*pelian*) rites is commonly articulated by the otherwise eager audience. This, however, should not be misunderstood, for deception in the material reality, as opposed to the corresponding reality of the dead, whose existence is a replica of that of the living, is in fact a demonstration of the great skill of the *manang*.

> Simulation is the hallmark of the *manang's* action in this world and the curative force of his actions in the other world. This is an entirely appropriate weapon to use against spirits who epitomize dangerous duplicity. In the end, the *manang* out-deceives the arch-deceiver by sheer artifice (Barrett, 1993: 268).

Cultural conditioning is not easily rooted out, and when these include processes of inclusion of individuals that would in a Western context be subject to severe marginalisation, culture may act as a protective factor for vulnerable individuals. In this study certain ethnic groups at Hospital Tranquillity are both over- and under-represented, a subject that is discussed in greater detail in Chapter Eight. A complex and ambiguous interplay of ideologies can be identified between psychiatric diagnosis and cultural constructs, where the nature and cause of the affliction, coupled with the degree of social disorder created and the means for restoration, may have an enormous impact on how well individuals interpret and overcome their own crises. As Warner points out:

> This may explain why even those individuals who are treated in modern Western-style hospitals and clinics in the developing world rather than by indigenous therapists may experience a higher recovery rate from psychosis (Warner, 1996: 61).

This suggests that the role of the traditional healer cutting across ethnic boundaries appears to be a pivotal issue in attempting to understand the cultural dynamics that revolve around sickness and cure in a multiethnic community. The degree of competition between the diverse healing specialisms remains unclear in this context. Nonetheless this intriguing situation raises the question of how, if at all, cultural processes may be beneficial to the individual, even when they stand beyond the direct support of the specific culture context.

Lenore Manderson (1996) in discussing the Malayan region of the nineteenth century in general, asserts that like modern practitioners in Malaysia, colonial authorities were usually tolerant towards plural medicine. Arguing that for the colonial powers this removed responsibility from the authorities, which could then continue to rest with the local communities (Manderson, 1996). Writing in the mid-twentieth century, Nissom and Schmidt (1967) used local Bidayuh folklore to suggest that amongst this populous Dayak group mental illness has traditionally been regarded as rare, unavoidable and virtually predestined with few precautions available, other than the observation of *patang* (taboo) rules. Schmidt (1964) further claimed that the importance of traditional healers in dealing with mental illnesses should therefore not be underestimated and, commensurate with Manderson's argument, should be viewed with tolerance.

> As mental health workers in other parts of the world, it has become clear to us in Sarawak also, that native healers play an important part in the treatment especially of mental illness. They have done so successfully for centuries before modern scientific psychiatry ever came to the Sarawak scene (Schmidt, 1964: 150).

Yet with regards to nineteenth-century Borneo it would be untrue to assume that the colonial authorities were complacent about leaving health care to local practitioners and they appear at times to have made strenuous efforts at times to improve health. Dr. A.W. Nieuwenhuis, a Dutch physician in Western Borneo from 1891-1901, described the scourge of malaria, smallpox, cholera and other virulent epidemics, which badly affected the local population in geographical pockets. Influenza, dysentery, skin diseases and notoriously syphilis, the unwelcome by-product of exposure to colonial trade, also took a heavy toll in terms of morbidity and mortality. Successful treatment, according to the author, assured good relationships towards the foreigners, facilitating compliance towards imperial rule, and to paraphrase Manderson (1996: 231) reinforcing the 'moral authority' and superiority of Western science over indigenous paradigms.

> Treatment with antisyphilitica often gave striking results, pains which had been felt for years being relieved and finally cured. This undoubtedly contributed in just as great a degree as the distribution of quinine, towards winning the confidence of the Dayak tribes of Central Borneo in the Europeans, and towards making my scientific trips a success (Nieuwenhuis, 1929: 16)

Whilst the benevolent 'scientific European, as representative of his civilisation', was engaged in dispensing *free* and *modern* health care, Nieuwenhuis spares no pains in drawing a contrast between European science and local charlatans amongst the Malay and Chinese selling 'quack medicines' to the ingenuous Dayak to assure themselves 'of an excellent source of income'[4] (Nieuwenhuis, 1929: 33).

During the nineteenth century the low and even falling population density of Borneo was noted with concern by the colonial powers as an anomalous situation compared to the rest of the region that threatened to deplete the labour force available to them (Knapen, 1997). Knapen (1997, 1998) records that consequently the authorities suggested with disapproval that this was probably due the assumed practice of infanticide. Or even to Dayak women's renowned expertise with birth control, rather than through the series of natural and human-caused disasters that plagued the region. Floods and droughts caused widespread destruction as did epidemics, while warfare and headhunting combined with power play and struggles for dominance amongst local and colonial forces contributed to large-scale social upheaval (Knapen, 1997). Although the death toll was very high amongst local populations, the colonial presence was also very badly affected by disease, as were indeed other migrants including the Chinese (Chew, 1990).

Knapen (1997; 1998) goes on to say that trade and expansion of the region economically over the centuries was seen by local populations as the main culprit in the introduction and spread of epidemics from increased contact with Europeans, Javanese traders and other non-indigenous groups keen to exploit the wealth of the island[5]. So associated with disease were foreign traders that many Dayak villages took the precaution of extreme isolation to protect themselves from epidemics as well as involvement in local warfare and head trophy taking.

> The only option which the Borneans had was to isolate themselves by declaring their villages forbidden territory, closing off rivers with rattan cords or tree trunks, excluding those infected from the village, fencing in their houses or, as a last resort, fleeing or migrating upriver. Nomadic groups like the Punan, of course, had much less trouble isolating themselves from the outside world. There are even indications of their practice of 'silent barter' (as being) a consequence of recurrent epidemics (Knapen, 1997: 127).

Evidently the great uncertainties of life instilled locals with a deep fear of epidemics and, understandably, of foreigners as well. Expansion and advancing 'civilisation' brought in its wake the loss of traditional methods of controlling disease while increasing the number of epidemics, and accelerating their growth to remote populations (Knapen, 1998). Although acknowledging the psychological strains of these traumatic changes Nieuwenhuis, followed eventually by Schmidt (1964), ascribes anxieties amongst Dayak groups as a consequence of the benighted superstitions of individuals at the mercy of forces they could not control.

(Dayaks) Probably suffered more psychologically than physically and have therefore become extremely afraid of their natural surroundings ... Like many other tribes they ascribe this to an army of spirits which they imagine exist in all prominent places. Misfortunes, disease and adversity are regarded as punishments inflicted by these spirits at the command of the chief god, for offences committed on earth. Influenced by this conviction, they have developed their *pantang* system (taboo rules) and foretoken belief until it dominates their lives (Nieuwenhuis, 1929: 26)

Epidemics and natural disasters combined with the low population interfered with the expansion plans brought by the colonial powers. The background to the *enlightened* medical care, which physicians like Nieuwenhuis brought to Borneo from Europe, camouflages the economic interests that the Dutch had vested in exploration and colonisation. The imperialistic expansion of the Dutch found a counterpart in the equally determined expansion of the British Empire, using similar tactics of paternalistic and benign medicine as envoys of peaceful intent and civilising rule. Manderson, however, identifies the liberal offering of European health care towards indigenous people as intimately connected with vested economic interests of Empire building.

Medicine is exposed as participating in the expansion and consolidation of political rule through its service to political, commercial and military arms of empire, leading to campaigns to conquer diseases that threatened the integrity and economic potentiality of the state, and to the systemic delivery of sanitary, health care and medical services (Manderson, 1996: 5).

In Borneo, Knapen (1979), for instance, comments on the Dutch attempts to actively suppress headhunting out of humanitarian and economic concerns, a similar move to that carried out by James Brooke on the other side of the island. Similarly, epidemics caused not only death but also the full-scale evacuation of people from their homes, much to the despair of colonial plantation owners who were reliant on local labour (Knapen, 1979: 2).

It would seem from these accounts that the main preoccupation, in the Borneo region at least, was the exposure of communities to virulent epidemics with further repercussions brought by political domination, debt slavery, localised warfare and trophy head-hunting taking a toll on the security of besieged communities. The prevalence of mental illness amongst individuals is uncertain and little remarked upon in accounts, but it is likely to have held a low priority as a health issue compared to the physical hazards that seem to have been a yearly event, in which women and children were considered to be the most vulnerable to the psychological strains of uncertainty and fear (Nieuwenhuis, 1929: 26). The local population would remain unacquainted with the trappings of civilised colonial rule in the shape of asylum care until the twentieth century when Sarawak boasted of its first psychiatric institution in the 1920s under the latter days of the Brooke dynasty.

The demise of the 'therapeutic' asylum in pre and post-war Malaya

Prior to World War II three further psychiatric institutions were built following the example of the Central Mental Hospital in Perak. In 1933 the State of Johore, a sultanate under British suzerainty, established first of all a lunatic asylum and in 1935 a psychiatric hospital to absorb the overspill of admissions. In the Borneo States of Sarawak and Sabah, two further hospitals were built in the period leading up to the 1950s (Tan and Wagner, 1971: 6-7). By the Second World War the huge numbers of admissions had severely compromised the quality of care in asylums:

> The concept that mental hospitals were asylums first and hospitals second probably led to the centralisation of facilities and huge catchment areas covering hundreds of miles. Thus patients with mental illnesses were transported by trains with escorts from all over the country ... The separation from families and its ill effects as well as that of long stay were not seen as problems (Deva, 1992: 500).

Finally, Woon (1971) records a dark hour for Malaya's psychiatric care following the invasion of the country by Japanese troops during World War II and the subsequent retreat of the British and Australian forces (1971). In the cities looting and anarchy reigned, with a skeleton staff remaining to care for the patient population nonetheless. The death rate for patients caused by abandonment, starvation and gross neglect was enormous. In Singapore many psychiatric patients starved to death after being abandoned on the small island of St John's to fend as best they could, following the requisitioning of their psychiatric hospital facilities by the Japanese occupying forces (Ng and Chee, 2006). In turn, Woon (1971) estimates that 3,800 patients alone died at the asylum at Tanjong

Rambutan, Ipoh under Japanese occupation, and many female patients were kidnapped with, no doubt, grim results for there is no record of their safe return (Woon, 1971).

Following the war the asylums were once more inundated with patients overwhelming the disproportionately few staff. In contrast with the dedicated improvement that had taken place in the past, the condition of the Central Mental Hospital, Perak, for instance, was rife with incompetence and malpractice (Tan and Wagner, 1971), a situation by no means unusual in British asylums of this period either, as has been attested by former inmates (Bell, 1996; Laing, 1996). These institutional abuses in Malaya indirectly led to a Royal Commission of Inquiry in 1957, and resulted in the discovery of various forms of malpractice taking place in the rigid hierarchy of asylum care. The culmination of these inquiries led to further investigations and recommendations for improvements by the World Health Organisation in 1960 (Deva, 1992; Deva, 1995).

By the time of Sarawak's accession to the Federation of Malaysia, apart from the four government-run hospitals, Hospital Bahagia (Perak), Hospital Permai Tampoi (Johore), Bukit Padang (Sabah) and the Sarawak Mental Hospital, there began a move away from large, centralised asylum care towards community-based care reflecting a global trend and a new level of optimism (Busfield, 1996b; Campbell, 1996; Caplan and Caplan, 2000; Deva, 2004). The National Community Mental Health Programme, introduced in 1996, has been at the forefront of training frontline staff, supported by institutional links with Britain (Deva, 2004). Decentralisation has to-date resulted in the development of several small psychiatric units in general hospitals which now number nearly a score. In addition there are now over 80 community-based psychiatric clinics spread unevenly over the country and in Sarawak, although generally regarded as less developed than Peninsular Malaysia, services do not compare unfavourably with those of the mainland. Yet, despite the gradual growth of psychiatric resources in Malaysia, the number of psychiatrists has been woefully low with a serious shortage in relation to the recommendation by the World Health Organization (WHO) which states that there should be a ratio of 1:100,000. The exact number of psychiatrists has been in dispute, however, it appears that at the turn of the millennium the total number was under 105, but it is known that in Sarawak the ratio was closer to 1:270,000 with less than half of these psychiatrists in government-run practice (Ashencaen Crabtree and Chong, 2001). Additionally the number of supporting health professionals has been correspondingly low, with few trained psychiatric nursing staff and even fewer psychiatric social workers

(Ashencaen Crabtree and Chong, 2001). This evidently indicates that this is an area of care that does not attract skilled and qualified candidates in sufficient numbers

Nursing and social work are professions stereotypically associated with women in industrialised societies like Britain and Malaysia. Consequently, insights developed in relation to professional work and gender in this area holds relevance for both countries through historical ties and economic similarities (Carter *et al.*, 1992; Dominelli, 1992). Gittins, for example, notes that in the 1920s psychiatric nursing was seen as a considerably less attractive option for women than it was for male attendants, who found compensations in the 'perks' of the job, such as security, cheap lodging and free uniforms, in comparison with exposure to the exigencies of a depressed post-war economy (Gittins, 1998: 114). Many of these difficulties have not been resolved over time, however, and in contemporary Britain concerns are expressed that psychiatric nursing retains an unappealing profile and continues to be bedevilled by staffing problems that of necessity impact on patient care (Hatfield *et al.*, 1992). Noteworthy areas of concern lie in the 'burn-out' and demoralisation of staff working in a 'culture of blame' (SNMAC, 1999: 18). Other difficulties include the managing of a heterogeneous and demanding patient population in an increasingly custodial and occasionally violent environment (Gostin, 1986). Once again, trends in Britain can be seen to be mirrored in the findings in the study, in which the views of staff at Hospital Tranquillity towards such issues as personal risk and career opportunities are considered in juxtaposition with the perspectives of patients.

Finally, the development of psychiatric services in Malaya, and to a lesser degree Borneo, can be viewed as not only running a parallel course to that taking place in Britain throughout most of its history, but also as having been directly predicated upon its examples. The introduction, for instance, of the asylum as therapeutic and basically benevolent foreshadowed its deterioration as a vast and dehumanising warehouse of neglected inmates. Furthermore, European attitudes towards ethnicity and gender informed psychiatric values and practices in colonised regions. Up to the present time the training of Malaysian-born psychiatrists has largely been undertaken in the West and philosophies of pathology, care and management frequently imported wholesale to the homeland (Deva, 2004). These approaches have then been applied to an ethnically diverse population, culturally removed from the European context in which psychiatry first emerged. Thus, it is argued, perpetuating the colonialism in postcolonial nations and thereby inhibiting the use and rediscovery of indigenous methods (Fernando, 2010).

The psychiatric service user experience, has developed from a radical ideological shift in the ownership of discourse where until comparatively recently, the voices of psychiatric patients were overridden by the infinitely more powerful messages of the medical elite. In Malaysia service user narratives remain an area that is shrouded in obscurity and poorly researched in general, particularly those of inpatients in psychiatric institutions; while patient accounts from the past appear to be so rare as to be effectively non-existent (Porter, 2006).

Although 'service user' voices are a rarity in historical accounts of psychiatric services - assuming for one moment that the conceptualised ideology inherent in this term carries any relevance in reference to past eras – these remain almost equally obscured for contemporary Malaysian psychiatric users. The following chapter, however, introduces the reader to the social and spatial context of Hospital Tranquillity, in which participant voices emerge to describe the ontological realities of lives subsumed under the self-perpetuating system of the asylum.

Notes

1   Authenticisation refers to professional practice that is grounded in the cultural schema and knowledge base of ethnic groups, over and above the adaptations of indigenisation (Baba et al, 2010; Ling, 2007).

2   Barrett draws out the distinction between the differing traditions in American and British social anthropology, in which for the latter, the term 'spirit medium' is a more familiar one, although both tend to draw a distinction between this role and that of priest (Barrett, 1993: xx-xxi).

3   The combining of these two distinctive academic subjects is not unknown amongst academics writing of Asian communities, as exemplified in particular by Arthur Kleinman's works.

4   Coastal Malay practitioners gained control over effective forms of treatment, such as variants of vaccination introduced by eighteenth-century Chinese or possibly the later Dutch, which used exposure techniques to the pus or skin crusts of infected smallpox patients. Malay practitioners notoriously charged local Dayak people exorbitant amounts for this uncertain treatment (Knapen, 1998).

5   Although trade expanded in the Borneo region considerably between the seventeenth and nineteenth centuries, the local population of Borneo has always relied on trade for essential and luxury items. Some of the most exciting

artefacts traded vigorously between the twelfth and eighteenth centuries were ceramic ware from China, Vietnam and Thailand, these being highly coveted items for their practical and decorative possibilities (Harrison, B. (1991) *Pusaka, Heirloom Jars of Borneo*. Oxford University Press: Singapore.

4

The transformation to patient-hood

Hospital Tranquillity occupies an ambiguous position in public perceptions in that primarily it embodies in concrete form the connotations of stigma that mental illness represents in Malaysia (Lau and Hardin, 1996; Trad, 1991; Wintersteen *et al.*, 1997). At the same time it attempts to counteract this image through public-relation exercises aimed at informing the general public, resulting in exhibitions, public talks and media statements. The hospital's appearance works to its advantage in this endeavour, as it is not unattractive and is far less forbidding than many of the Gothic psychiatric establishments built in nineteenth-century Britain, as epitomised by the gigantic London County Asylum at Colney Hatch (Shorter, 1997). Literally and metaphorically this appearance is a misleading façade for many of the practices and attitudes found at the hospital have long roots that are firmly grounded in traditional asylum care.

These days one enters Hospital Tranquillity via a long drive and then through a main door that is decorated with floral murals. One is then presented with the view of a long, low, whitewashed quadrangle of administrative offices, open-plan wards and recreational workshops built around a central square lawn. Two long arms of corridors extend at the end of this contained quadrangle that lead, at the time of the study, to the private wing, and at the other end to the general wards. The long drive to the hospital, its high walls and long corridors are a miniaturised reflection of the established Victorian institution design in creating a sense of seclusion from the community, as well as forming practical means for the easy surveillance of patients (Jones, 1993). In this way the layout of the hospital typifies a fundamentally pragmatic if value-laden design reminiscent of Saris' descriptions of the ideal asylum, albeit on a much reduced scale (Saris, 1996).

In keeping with the contemporary health system in Malaysia, as well as traditional asylum care which catered to private patients as well as paupers, class differentials are carefully built into the geographic space of the hospital. Fee-paying first- and second-class wards have been based at one end of the

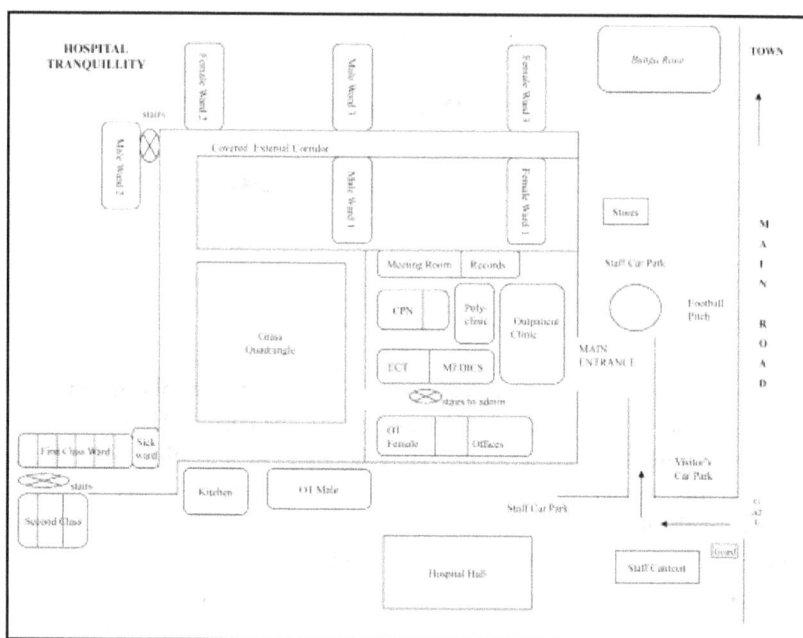

hospital in a pleasant area of brightly planted containers, and to reach the single-bedroom units of the first-class wards the visitor is obliged to walk uphill to a small oasis of greenery. By contrast, the majority of the congested non-paying 'public' wards are reached by walking in the opposite direction heading downhill. More recently, and presumably owing to overcrowding issues on the public wards, some long stay male patients have been permitted into the more spacious and little used private grounds.

In common with many British hospitals of the same era, the hospital is also segregated by sex with men and women occupy exclusive spaces, reinforcing notions of gender difference and the presumed hazards and attractions of mixing freely with the opposite sex (Clark, 1996; Gittins, 1998). In this vein Foucault draws a somewhat abstract observation of psychiatric institutions,

(With their) large populations, their hierarchies, their spatial arrangements, their surveillance systems (these are) delineated areas of extreme sexual saturation (Foucault, 1976b: 46).

As Foucault conveys, this segregation serves to conspicuously underline the very issues of sexuality and gender that such spatial strategies attempted to evade in the first place. Furthermore, just as men are firmly separated from women at Hospital Tranquillity, there exists a further category of men who are separated from their own sex. These are the men of *Bunga Raya* ward - a place that stands apart from the rest of the hospital, in an isolated block. This is the forensic ward where the criminally insane are housed. It has no female counterpart in this hospital and is a unique environment, one that is both a part of, and yet stands apart from the rest of the hospital. A pervading air of notoriety and danger is associated with *Bunga Raya*, which deters most visitors, and female staff rarely enter there unless accompanied by an escort.

As indicated in reference to Saris (1996) the spatial and metaphysical aspects of psychiatric institutions have increasingly become a topic of academic inquiry, in which social scientists explore both the geography of such environments and their implicit meanings for inhabitants, and the general public alike. Parr and Philo (1996), for example, analyse historical British asylums in terms of literal and moral space – the environmental context where a certain ethos and value base is played out. Another useful perspective is offered by Phyllis Montgomery (2001: 426-427), who follows Soja (1996) in viewing the institution in terms of a 'plurality of space' that incorporates three inter-related spaces. These are described as 'firstspace', 'secondspace' and 'thirdspace' respectively, and are defined as firstly relating to the physical, concrete context. Next, that which is identified space and mapped for a purpose; and finally, *thirdspace* relates to the lived experience of those who use such spaces, rescuing their voices for inclusion as an additional dimension of the phenomena.

These three aspects are explored in-depth here, the narratives of patients and staff emerging from, and providing crucial insights into the material environment and the rules that govern it.

Categorising patients: The 'salvageable' and the 'irredeemable'

The 'acute' wards for male and female patients were originally visible from each other as dormitory blocks separated by high chain-linked grounds. Such has been the symmetry of the wards that public wards at ground level are placed one behind the other across a partially covered corridor. The major part of fieldwork was spent on these two wards which are still, in comparison with the 'chronic' wards, relatively busy environments, and where the small but resident long-stay population of the acute wards is varied by a background of admissions and discharges of first-admission and multiply admitted patients.

While staff used the terms 'acute' and 'chronic' with the matter-of-fact attitude of those comfortable with accepted definitions, I was unclear about what was meant in each case. Consequently I questioned staff on most wards about how *they* used this term and which patients might be considered acute and which chronic. The outcome of this line of questioning was insightful, but nonetheless raised more questions than answers. Fifty-five year old Margot, a Chinese woman on Female Ward 2, who, I knew well, would be classified as a chronic patient, had lived at Tranquillity since being admitted as an unruly teenager. Despite her years, Margot emanated innocence under siege. A gentle individual, with a rather childlike and indeed naïve air about her, she endured the rough and tumble of hospital life by hiding from aggressors and seeking out sympathetic companions among the staff and visitors like myself, or withdrawing into a distancing state of muteness, in which at times she seemed utterly lost. An extract from field notes provides a thumbnail sketch of Margot and the kinds of interaction we experienced when Margot was feeling cheerful and well.

Field notes: Female Ward 2.

Saw Margot who was as usual carrying round a child's bucket filled with an odd assortment of items that represent her worldly possessions. Margot was feeling friendly and wanted to chat. Once again, I tried to get a coherent story out of her without luck, and had to rely on the broken threads of narrative she offered that were picked up and dropped at short intervals. Fortunately among the verbal flotsam- and jetsam were interesting clues to be turned over and mulled at leisure. A sociable person by nature Margot, however, is often lost in forlorn, confused thoughts about her former family, with many anxieties about 'misbehaving'.

Today I discovered that her name is an alias. In fact, as a Chinese woman she carries a Chinese name and she was given the nickname of 'Margot' by an aunt due to her childhood love of dancing - a *veritable* Margot Fonteyn. Margot doesn't do much dancing these days though, and sometimes I come across her in a frozen posture, apparently unable to speak at all. Today she is also preoccupied by her need to 'talk, talk, talk', for which apparently she has been scolded by nurses in OT. This is very sad, as when she feels well Margot is an animated and charming person, which stands in contrast to the mute and utterly bewildered figure on the ward at other times

In her study of psychiatric service users attending a community-based service in Wisconsin, Sue Estroff (1985: 44) notes that the term 'chronicity' is generally used to define the duration of illness, but is also used in relation to 'psychiatric, social, behavioral, attitudinal and interpersonal characteristics'. An individual such as Margot would probably be seen as a typical example of the chronic patient in her inability to communicate her thoughts adequately, combined with her obsessions, her odd habits and peculiar appearance. Roger Gomm suggests that 'chronicity' is more generally used to describe the effects of 'institutionalisation': the petrifaction of individuals into a 'mental illness role', and again Margot would appear to fit this description as well on her 'bad' days (Gomm, 1996: 81).

At Tranquillity, staff found it fairly difficult to precisely pinpoint the nature of 'chronicity' but described it in terms of practical considerations governing classification in a somewhat nebulous and circuitous way. To clarify the explanation then, on the 'acute wards' Female Ward 1 and Male Ward 1 the tempo is livelier and 'acute' patients are regarded as being in certain ways 'salvageable'. Once they are no longer suffering from a psychosis or any other condition affecting orientation or lucidity, patients on these wards are more likely to be responsive to visitors such as myself, and are therefore popular places for visiting nursing students and doctors. On these wards, multiply admitted 'acute' patients form the largest group. Some veterans have been admitted on scores of occasions spanning decades in a 'revolving-door' cycle, managing nonetheless to avoid a permanent admission, almost always due to continued family support in the community.

Once this family support is seen to fail, however, and patients spend longer and longer periods at the hospital, their status becomes redefined, even though their actual diagnosis may remain unchanged. Eventually this may lead to the new, demoted classification of the irredeemable 'chronic' patient, with an entirely different level of professional expectation attached to their condition. The point at which practical hope is lost that a patient can be discharged back to the family 'home', is seen as a significant turning-point, where a patient is transformed into a 'chronic' patient, and an almost inevitable downward path is charted, from which only a rare occurrence can prevent permanent custodial care and exile from life beyond the hospital walls.

This general description, rather than specific identification, conforms more closely to Arthur Kleinman's discussion of the term in which,

Chronicity is not simply a direct result of pathology acting in an isolated person. It is the outcome of lives lived under constraining circumstances with particular relationships to other people. Chronicity is created in part out of negative expectations that come to be shared in face-to-face interactions – expectations that fetter out dreams and sting and choke our sense of self (Kleinman, 1988a: 180).

Chronic patients at Tranquillity therefore are those who have been hospitalised without discharge for years on end. Viewed as hopelessly 'institutionalised', regardless of the status of their illness, they are seen as incapable of surviving outside of custodial care without family support. This stands in direct contrast to the defined status of 'acute' patients who can and do survive beyond the walls of the hospital.

The incarceration and waste of potential of so-called chronic patients is not unappreciated by the staff on the wards, who refer to the plight of their human flotsam in various emotive ways. I repeatedly heard of chronic patients being described by staff as having been 'dumped' and 'abandoned' to hospital care, as a further extract from field notes illustrates.

Field notes: Male Ward 3.

The staff seem pleased to see me on the whole, and they are friendly and interesting; perhaps they are suffering from boredom. They show me one hapless Chinese patient of around 30- or 40-years-old with wasted, bent limbs, curled up on a plastic chair, and cheerily show me his case file. 'He's a rich man!' An MA (medical assistant) bursts out. 'Yes, a rich man. His father owned many acres and died leaving it to him, but then the uncle took it because he (the patient) is a mental sub (mentally subnormal). But the hospital said he (uncle) must pay for 2nd class for this fellow, so at least he gets something. He doesn't have to be here – he could go home if someone feeds him with a spoon, but no they don't want him at home, so he must stay here.'

In the opinion of the staff, therefore, chronic patients are victims not so much of society, their illnesses or a psychiatric system that fails to find alternative means of care, but of uncaring families, who are seen to be abrogating their duty to take care of their mentally ill relative for life (Ashencaen Crabtree, 2001).

In this regard, the position of patients at Tranquillity is not dissimilar to counterparts in the traditional asylum system in Britain, for instance, where family support was pivotal to any possible hope of discharge, given the almost total lack of appropriate resources in society. Although community resources are by no means as entirely absent in a modern-day Malaysian

State, these are, as yet, still not able to offer the support to patients sufficient to extricate the majority from long years spent in institutional care.

Finally, since a large majority of inpatients at Tranquillity are long-stay individuals there were four times as many general wards for the chronically ill as there were for acute cases. Quite a few long-stay veterans on the acute wards are destined in due course for the chronic wards. While they can cope adequately and are youthful and active in most respects, they will stay on the acute wards for as long as possible.

The years in institutional care often leave an indelible mark on psychiatric patients, which militated against my overtures to develop a conversational relationship. For many such patients, like Margot, it was not possible to maintain a conversation long enough for me to be able to extract a coherent account from the fragments of information seemingly arbitrarily strewn. This said, my presence could be greeted with enthusiasm by patients on some of the wards, particularly Female Ward 2 and Male Ward 2, which either by design or accident were home to a fairly gregarious set of people eager to shake hands and say hello, even when little that could be gleaned was deeply illuminating. Under these circumstances, it was not the verbal responses but my observation of the every-day behaviour of patients and staff and the routines implemented and submitted to, that provided most of my understanding of what the chronic wards were like to live on.

The cycle of patient-hood through admission and discharge

In interview it was often quite difficult to obtain much insight into how patient respondents perceived their admissions. Most had been openly escorted by family or through some form of guile, while some had been admitted by the police under dramatic and often traumatic circumstances. Although respondents normally indicated an awareness of a transgression somewhere, this was not usually discussed in specific terms. Rather it remained a vague and uncertain set of circumstances, although some, of both sexes, admitted that violence or destruction of property had initiated action. Dimbaud, a muscular and handsome Dayak man, was amused to describe his first admission to hospital. Smiling broadly, cradling an adopted, scrawny stray kitten in his arms, he vigorously described a frightening psychotic and aggressive episode, in which much furniture was demolished, with fortunately few injuries inflicted, following a prolonged bout of drinking *langkau* (an extremely powerful and toxic 'moonshine'). His tale is a reminder of how acohol abuse was also considered sufficient cause for enforced admission to asylum care in the past, along with other manifestations of social problems.

Newcomer Ai Lan, a limply passive and depressed young woman on her first admission, was propped in an upright chair, blankly recounting how she had threatened to kill a member of her family in a family row before turning her aggression on herself in an abortive attempt to drown herself in the river. Based on feminist critiques that claim a preponderance towards female admission to psychiatric services universally, my initial assumption on commencing fieldwork was predictably, that this would prove to be the situation at Hospital Tranquillity as well (Chesler, 1996; Russell, 1995; Wetzel, 2000). Contrary to my expectations however, statistical records from Hospital Tranquillity suggested that a significant bias towards the admission of women over and beyond that of men may not be the general trend. Available statistics from the hospital were usually not up-todate but based on retrospective records, at least a couple of years old in many instances. Nonetheless these statistics revealed that admission figures broken down into gender variables over a two-year 'snapshot' of admissions, demonstrated that the sexes were fairly equally represented during this time, with a slight bias towards men. In 1997, for example, men represented 57% of multiple admissions (defined effectively as anyone on their second and subsequent admission) at Hospital Tranquillity and by 1998 the number had risen slightly to 58% of all admissions. Additionally in 1997 men still outnumbered women in terms of first admissions by a ratio of 68% but by 1998 this had dropped to 62%. Evidently, for this particular hospital during this brief historical period at least, and in keeping with historical accounts of colonial asylums, women patients were not admitted in higher numbers to those of men (Ernst, 2010). Instead, the sexes appeared to occupy an equal footing in terms of diagnosis and custodial care, albeit that the reasons given for admission did not reveal a gender-neutral territory.

By 2008, statistics were no longer transparent or openly available and far more difficult to obtain through formal request. This was in turn a reflection of how difficult access to hospital information had become; several psychiatric hospitals, previously willing to share such information, were now operating tightly restrictive access to researchers, nationals and foreigners, for reasons that remain unknown. However, what data was made available in 2008 indicates that at Hospital Tranquility the figures for inpatients across gender indicate that men are overrepresented across wards by a varying rate running close to 15%.

Patients under compulsory admission orders are usually brought to Tranquillity under an antiquated piece of legislation built on the foundations of colonial legislation, which has remained in a virtually static state in independent Malaysia. This legislation is known as the 'Mental Health Ordinance Sarawak 1961' and like its UK counterpart, the Mental Health Act 1983, the Mental Health Ordinance Sarawak 1961 states that compulsory admission to hospital can only be made in order to protect the patient or others from harm. However, there is an added clause that states that admission can be undertaken on the grounds of the protection of property from damage by the patient.

The Sarawak legislation does not offer a definition of mental illness, unlike the UK 1983 Act, but refers to mental illness or mental 'defect' as being of an 'unsound mind'. Consequently no distinction is made between mental disorders, illnesses and learning disabilities. That this *does* mean that detention at the hospital is made of people with epilepsy, Down's Syndrome, and other disabilities loosely categorised as 'mentally subnormal', is made apparent through statistical data pertaining to Hospital Tranquillity. This, however, is quite in keeping with the history of psychiatry, where extraordinarily diverse population of patients were held in asylums from the late 1860s onwards, having moved from providing care for seriously mentally disturbed people, to being vast communes accommodating virtually anyone perceived to be a burden or inconvenience to their family, society or themselves; adding, needless to say, to the exponential growth of detainees (Murphy, 1991; Scull, 1993).

Finally, in Sarawak the process of admittance empowers a magistrate to order the apprehension of 'any person reported to be of an unsound mind or to be behaving in such a manner as to suggest that he is of unsound mind' for a period not 'exceeding one calendar month' (Mental Health Ordinance Sarawak No. 16, 1961: 4 (2.1): 2), at which time a medical report must be prepared and following this period an inquiry held. However as the Act goes on to say, the detainee has no right to be present at an inquiry if the Magistrate 'is satisfied that, by reason of his lack of understanding, no good purpose would be served by his attendance' (No. 16, 1961: 9 (1): 3).

By comparison to contemporary Britain the Approved Mental Health Professional (formerly known as the Approved Social Worker) social work role is premised upon the need to preserve the rights of psychiatric patients in admission procedures, and while this is in the process of revision, a corresponding role has never evolved in the Malaysian system (Butler and Pritchard, 1983; Hudson, 1982; Pringle and Thompson, 1986). Heavy paternalism has tended to dominate proceedings in the admittance of patients in Sarawak and once in custody of care the coordination and the statutory observation of the processes of admittance and review can frequently be haphazard. According to a prominent official overseeing psychiatric services it has not been uncommon for the maximum period of confinement to be overlooked by busy staff or unconcerned relatives.

> *(Compulsory) Certification to hospital is currently unstandardised throughout the country, which is a problem. A more rapid admission procedure is also needed as currently this all goes through a magistrate .... And furthermore protection of patients' rights needs to be looked at. The current situation, especially in Sarawak, is that a family can have a patient compulsorily admitted against their will, and even against the medical opinion of a doctor, who may feel that they can be cared for as an out-patient. These admissions usually take place under section 13, of the Mental Health Ordinance '61, which is actually for temporary admissions only, but the time of detention is usually poorly monitored.*

Under this system, there has been no specific right to appeal, and the boundaries of voluntary and compulsory admission are blurred, whereby individual circumstances of admission and rights to discharge remain unclear to patients. The resulting situation is that all admissions act in effect as mandatory and indefinite periods of custodial care, in which patients are subjected to a forcible socialisation into conformity, without any professional or legal acknowledgement that they may legitimately, in the case of so-called voluntary admissions, 'opt out' or demand a review tribunal.

The long awaited Mental Health Act 2001 has gone through the Malaysian parliamentary process but has yet to fully implemented. This was originally viewed as superseding the Mental Health Ordinance Sarawak 1961, and two other pieces of anachronistic legislation: the Mental Health Disorder Ordinance 1956, and the evocatively named, Lunatic Ordinance of Sabah, 1953 (Ashencaen Crabtree and Chong, 2000). Within the revised Act there are a number of familiar formalities designed to safeguard the rights of individuals. These refer to a formal notification of detention in a psychiatric institution, together with a medical examination of a person's mental state within a 24-hour period of first detention. This cannot exceed a period of longer than one month without a further examination and case for detainment being made. Such precautions, duly enforced, may indeed ensure that the rights of individuals in institutional care are balanced more equally against the dominant voice of officialdom, and the weighty opinion of relatives, both of whom hold great authority over the lives of psychiatric service users in Malaysia. As yet, however, this remains a power balance that has yet to be tipped towards the latter, and is a long way from becoming more equalised.

In this vein, I had few opportunities to make a direct comparison of official rationales for admission compared with the views of patients on the subject. In general conversation with patient participants and staff, however, the views of the latter towards sanctioned professional intervention were often discordant with how patients saw their lives and hospitalisation – an experience that ex-psychiatric patients in the West have also claimed (O'Hagan, 1996).

These accounts from patients resonated with some of the theoretical positions of the so-called 'sociology of deviance', whereby transgressions of social norms are controlled through the labelling of transgressors as 'mentally ill' (Scheff, 1996: 65). To this well-known point, the 'myth' of mental illness, became a convenient way of pigeonholing the troubles of the poor, the excluded and the oppressed in society (Szasz, 1974). Labelling individuals as mentally ill thereby serves to compound the perceived problems in living (Gomm, 1996; Rosenhan, 1993). Goffman, in accord with Scheff, describes the 'moral career' of the psychiatric patient once labelled, as one of continuous professional discrediting of the patient's social self and mortification of their integrity (Goffman, 1993).

In this way, the narratives of patient participants could be seen to be accounts of life problems. These problems were seen as part of the individual's pathology and were then reframed as representational delusions and obsessions, confirming to staff, if need be, the diagnosis of mental infirmity. The original problems of individuals, grounded in gender stereotypes or in general poverty for instance, were obscured and distorted through the enforcement of the 'deviant role' of the psychiatric patient, as depicted in the following accounts (Scheff, 1976; Lemert, 1993a).

Abang was a multiply admitted, still youthful man on Male Ward 1 and although a reasonably capable individual was destined to join the legions of the 'chronic' eventually. The hospital represented an easy existence, one that he did not rail against and in fact seemed to have adapted to as a place of permanency. Neither perturbed nor particularly intrigued by my approach, he was willing to talk to me provided our discussion did not take up too much of his time. Consequently I learned that Abang's day revolved around sleep, meals, working in the occupational therapy unit, and, in particular, smoking; a description which once again mirrored the rigid pattern of 'sleep, work, eat, sleep' of the asylum regime (Murphy, 1991). This mundane existence was one he was resigned to living, as indeed he was equally resigned to describing, because his family had effectively consigned him to the care of the hospital on an indefinite basis, as he was seemingly unable to pull his weight at home and was evidently considered an expensive and dispensable liability.

> *It was my father who suggested I be here. He says I only eat and sleep at home but at least I can work here. If I am at home and suddenly my eyes roll up again I need to come back on that day itself. We don't really have enough money to pay for the bus fare. So since my father asked me to stay here I can work in the carpentry, I stay here, lah. Financially it is quite tight for my family and my father cannot afford to feed me. Besides, my father is a heavy smoker and he is old and cannot earn much.*

Poverty has often been linked with mental illness as a risk factor. Notably, however, in traditional, large asylums the vast majority of inmates were poor: either paupers to begin with or having become such through the repercussions of mental illness (Scull, 1993). For impoverished families, having to support unproductive relatives made the option of asylum care an obviously attractive one in relieving an unnecessary financial burden; a pragmatic equation that Abang's *kampung*-based father had duly calculated two hundred or so years later.

On the private ward Foo, a quiet, earnest and very anxious Chinese youth in his late twenties, regarded the hospital as a semi-voluntary retreat from the intolerable hurly-burly of life at home in the family-owned 'shop-house', to which he returned on 'home leave' every few weeks. Foo was preoccupied with guilt over his inability to help his widowed mother, for being the 'eldest son' in a Chinese family the expectations to shoulder the responsibilities undertaken by a head of the household would normally be very high. Consequently, his failure to do so was all the more painful. At home the pressure made him feel ill and quickly precipitated a semi-voluntary return to the undemanding environment of the private ward. His response would have been one entirely in keeping with the idealistic beliefs of early asylum proponents who regarded them as offering a therapeutic haven away from the undesirable influence of the patient's family and friends. On the other hand, for Foo, being in hospital was far from ideal. The ward 'has no freedom, the nurse there always direct you to do this and do that'. Foo considered the dilemma insoluable and concluded that it is better all round that he continued to regard the hospital as his real home with occasional, emotionally fraught visits back to the family home.

As physically fit young men Abang and Foo were socially expected to take up the role of main breadwinners and protectors of their family. A diagnosis of mental illness had prevented them from discharging these duties adequately and they were both now regarded as liabilities, to be discarded to an indefinite and emasculated exile at Tranquillity. For women patients at Tranquillity, however, their inability to meet socially expected obligations was perceived not in terms of being *de-sexed* by their incompetencies or as squanderers of limited resources, but rather as moral and sexual deviants, contaminators of the *status quo* and corrupters of their children (Barnes and Bowl, 2001: Cogliati *et al.*, 1988; Ussher, 1991).

The rates of fertility among psychiatric patients is lower than in the general population in the West, but gender demarcations exist in that there are far more women with psychiatric histories who are mothers, than male counterparts who are fathers (Diaz-Caneja and Johnson, 2004). In keeping with this phenomenon most men on Male Ward 1 were single men, whereas on Female Ward 1 many of the women there were mothers. Furthermore, these figures were also suggestive of the increased risk factors correlated with a diagnosis of mental illness and the state of maternity, as it is understood in the West (Ramon, 1996; Ussher, 1991).

These Malaysian women were understandably particularly traumatised by their diagnoses and admissions, with their thoughts continuously revolving around the welfare of their children, and for the most part were not resigned to their custody. Maria, a regular admission to the relative comfort of the private wards believed that 'stress' and a highly anxious, unassertive personality had deprived her of the opportunity of making more of a life. This was otherwise characterised by financial dependence on her husband and the trials of caring for her disabled child, as well as the loss of achieving her intellectual potential. Maria evidently missed her family a lot and telephoned them frequently, worrying considerably about her young child but feeling too overwhelmed to return home. Such was the stigma of her shameful inability to cope that her whereabouts were kept a secret from her child, who was duly told that his mother was away shopping on an indefinite and baffling spree.

Linda, like Maria, had been in and out of the hospital for years to the point that she now had no home left in the community. Ever dependent on a kind look or word, Linda mournfully enjoyed engaging my attention and pouring out a pitiful litany of sorrows. Linda usually talked about her lost son with palpable longing as she was forced to give up contact with him after her diagnosis and the consequential collapse of her marriage.

'I hasn't seen my son for seven years. I write so many letters asking photo. But he doesn't want to write to me... I went to my house when my boy was ten, but my husband he said 'don't speak to Mummy'. I think a woman was inside, his new woman...'

Elynna, a frantic young Iban woman and newly arrived first-admission patient, was appalled by her incarceration. Not long removed from the privileges of civil life she was outraged by her experiences and seemed very relieved to be able to talk about them to me. Recently brought 'unconscious' to the hospital (by which she meant an out-of-mind or psychotic state) after an attack of disorientation on the public street, Elynna recounted a tragic and typical tale of gender oppression and loss. Back in her village, her marriage failed when her husband left to eventually set up home with another woman and then refused to support his former family. Elynna took the bold step of later migrating to the city with her children in order to find work and while life continued to be hard for her, the family survived. One day, she says, her husband suddenly appeared and took the children from her, depositing them with one of her distant relatives, on the grounds that Elynna was earning a living as a prostitute, a common enough accusation levied against Iban women who take up a role solely designated for Iban male itinerants on *bejalai*[1]. This pejorative accusation was one that Elynna absolutely denied repeatedly to me as she had then. A year passed without her being allowed to see the children and to add to her injuries she was cast off by the rest of her family. Now forcibly hospitalised she was now distraught with worry and frustration, especially as she had been informed that there were moves afoot to formally adopt the children within the family against her wishes.

Elynna's narrative resonates with Jackson's (2005) discussion of the detention of African women in Southern Rhodesia by the colonial authorities, when found to be wandering beyond the home territory and away from their family. Such women were normally returned to the racially marginalised but apparent patriarchal authority of their husbands, by the complicit, colonial, institutionalised masculine hegemonic power (Connell, 1995); or otherwise admitted to the psychiatric hospital.

These sad narratives at Tranquillity, however, were not peculiar to the study participants by any means, but instead they hold a wider resonance regarding how madness in motherhood is perceived. The experiences of the Malaysian women here are echoed in accounts from female psychiatric service-users in Britain, for example. The loss of access to children is a devastating experience that is shared by many women across cultures, who have been thoroughly discredited as mothers by a diagnosis of mental illness (Jane, 1996: Ramon, 1996).

To return to the discharge process at Tranquillity, this, as in other hospitals, is reliant on the ward doctor's verdict, but without the option of voluntary discharge. For chronic patients, the lack of alternative facilities militates against their ever being able to achieve a discharge from hospital premises, and a similar situation exists on *Bunga Raya* ward. Ward staff pointed out one individual from an indigenous nomadic group now mandatorily 'resettled' by the Government for the purposes of a dam-building project. This man would, in all likelihood, remain permanently at the hospital despite his recent pardon from the State's Chief Minister, as his community had effectively exiled him for his crime of murder by refusing to accept him back. A return home to a hostile community struggling to survive a completely new way of life stacked the odds too heavily against success, in the opinion of the staff, who continued to hold him on the ward.

In general, hospital policies dictated that psychiatric patients needed to be discharged to the care of an escort, who was always a member of the family. Consequently, discharges were often delayed until such an escort was made available, and delays of hours, days, weeks and even years were by no means uncommon, as the following conversation indicates.

Field notes: Female Ward 1.

It's evening on the ward. The night shift has arrived on duty; they are sitting around taking a break while the ward settles down for the night. A young Chinese woman is anxiously asking the Sister in charge for permission to leave the ward to use the public telephone box at reception.

Patient:	I want to go out. I want to call home. My heart is like a rocket - I want to go home.
Nurse L:	How many times have you been out to telephone today? Five times? You stay on the ward now.
[Patient appeals to another nurse]	
Patient:	I want to go out to call my brother.
Nurse P:	You must listen to the Sister - if she says 'no' then *we* can do nothing.
Nurse L:	You've spoken to your brother, what did he say?
Patient:	He said that he had to ask my sister-in-law.
Nurse L:	What did she say?
Patient:	I didn't speak to her, only my brother. He said to wait, they would come later. But I want to call. Can I use the telephone here?
Nurse L:	No, that phone goes through to the operator. If they do not come by 9 o'clock, I will call them myself.

Patient:	I don't want this *baju* (hospital jacket) when I go home.
Nurse P:	You can wear your own *baju* - the yellow one you had when you came here.
Nurse L:	You wear that *baju* tonight and the yellow one to go home.
Nurse P:	You stay on the ward tonight. [Cajoling] One more night.
Patient:	Can I pay the hospital transport to take me home?
Nurse L:	No, the rules have changed. No transport. You would have to pay overtime.
Patient:	I want to call them.
Nurse L:	[Getting annoyed] You behave! You behave!
Nurse P:	One more night. Then you see the doctor tomorrow and he will decide for you.
Patient:	Can I go home then?
Nurse P:	Yes, a nurse can escort you - if you know the address. Where do you live?
[Patient hesitates over the address, nurses exchange a look]	
Nurse L:	[To me] She has been waiting all day to go home but no one has come to take her home yet. [To patient] Wait till tomorrow now – it's night-time now.
Researcher:	It must be very upsetting for her to wait for so long.
Nurse L:	[Aggrieved] She must not phone so much, they will think she is *still* ill. Once is enough.
[Patient gives up and wanders off.]	

The main assumption informing this general policy towards escorted discharge appeared to relate to the assumption that a psychiatric patient, and particularly a female patient, must remain under the custodial care of one carer or another. She is consequently not seen to be independent or autonomous by virtue of her recovery, and her discharge is therefore contingent on the cooperation of others, a situation which may cause a considerable amount of distress. While male patients are known to leave the hospital without an escort on occasions, and more often resort to 'absconding' given the opportunity, this level of independence is considered an unacceptable hazard in relation to women under hospital care. Consequently, patients in general, and women patients in particular, are expected to be entirely reliant on the coordination of families and staff to affect their discharge.

Ward life and the process of socialisation

Upon arrival at the hospital, probably the first thing that I noticed was the locked-up appearances of the four wards I had decided to focus on. Locked grill gates from the main corridors to the entrance of Female Wards 1 and 2, via their attached verandas, forced me to ask for permission to enter on nearly every occasion. My presence was virtually always spotted by one of the women patients who tended to hang around the gate peering at the occasional passer-by. She would then alert a nurse who would leisurely and elaborately unlock the large padlock on the door, permit me to enter, and then lock the gate up securely once again. The 'turn-key' operation was also in place on Male Ward 2, which, apart from *Bunga Raya* ward, was the most isolated on the hospital owing to its being the only ward located on a first floor. By contrast, there was usually free access to Male Ward 1, which was less often locked, and consequently had an air of being one of the most liberal wards. This, however, was belied by its formidable, overcrowded lock-up section, a feature of every public ward. However, it could be argued that at least there was company of a sort to be found in locked sections for both sexes. In some British psychiatric hospitals in the 1950s seclusion was routine, as for example was the case at Banstead Hospital in Surrey, later recalled by its former Deputy Superintendent, Dr A.A. Baker.

> Conditions were very bad there .... I was the only consultant on the female side which had 1,500 beds – seven wards of over 100 apiece, almost all of them locked ... .On the female side alone there were 50 or more patients who were secluded the whole day, some having been so for many months or even years at a stretch (Murphy, 1991: 53).

Due, seemingly to a fondness for symmetry, ward design at Hospital Tranquillity was very similar on the acute and chronic wards. On Female Ward 1, Male Ward 1 and Female Ward 2, a large veranda lead to the 'open ward' area flanked by the ward garden. On the verandas of Female Wards 1 and 2 were long trestle tables, often covered in plastic sheets, which were used for eating and general utility purposes, as well as work for the women patients. On Female Ward 1 large flower pots of camellias and bougainvillea were used for decorative effect, while in the latter months of fieldwork a small, rarely used badminton court was the main feature of the veranda area on Male Ward 1. The garden of Female Ward 2 was more utilitarian in appearance and graced with basic washing-up facilities of large plastic bowls, dish racks, scrubbing implements and a hose-pipe close to the view of passers-by. The veranda area of Male Ward 2 was the grimmest of all, being a balcony netted over with wire, lined with plastic chairs and with a floor littered with cigarette butts.

On these four wards, regardless of sex or duration of stay, the general appearance was one of sparseness, with an antiseptic quality created only in part by the smell of cleaning fluids, but mostly conveyed by the sheer bareness of the room and lack of decoration. The main ward on both units was a big open dormitory, where a dozen or so metal-framed hospital beds were lined against each of the longest walls, under the glassless, barred windows. At the far end of the ward was a barred and locked nursing room equipped with an examination bed, sinks and medicine units, where my interviews with patients were often conducted for want of a more conducive environment. At the other end of the room stood the 'locked' section, which was divided off from the rest of the 'open' ward by bars and acted as a self-contained unit, with its own beds for patients and a latrine.

By some of the beds on both 'open' wards an occasional, rickety bedside table was seen, but this was a rare piece of furniture, which on Male Ward 1 was often to be found with the drawer awkwardly pushed against the wall in an ineffectual attempt to deter theft, but making access a tricky business. Here there were practically no signs of the personal possessions of patients: no clothes or shoes in sight, no books, games or family photographs on view. Personal items were for the most part kept under the bed-mattresses for convenience, and these were usually items lacking in value, such as plastic sandals. Valuable items, primarily money, were safeguarded by the hospital authorities, and although the staff did assure me that patients could use security lockers for other possessions, I did not see evidence of patients using these during my visits, concluding that few possessions were brought into the ward upon admission.

Personalisation of space was made additionally problematic, in that although beds on the acute wards were nominally allocated to patients, they were in practice held in common, so that other patients might casually occupy beds as required. For some patients, particularly on Male Ward 1, this did not seem to overtly bother them. On Female Ward 1, however, the following rather fragmented discussion took place with Wei Hua, a young Chinese woman on her first admission, and Noor, a Malay 'old-hand', in which both women clearly express disgust at the communal bed practice due to the contamination of their sleeping areas by other patients who were voluntarily or involuntarily confined to bed.

Researcher: So, what do you think about sharing beds with other people here?

Wei Hua:	Sleeping ... the bed sheet (searches for word) ... blood... [makes a gesture indicating her vagina].
Researcher:	Period? Menstrual blood?
Noor:	Unclean.
Wei Hua:	And here [gestures towards her rump].
Researcher:	Faeces? Shit?
Wei Hua:	Don't like other people to sleep on your bed – smell.
Researcher:	So you cannot say, 'this is my bed'?
Noor:	No, they (the nurses) restrain people on beds – you cannot say 'this is my bed'.

For Noor and Wei Hua, the implication was that sleeping in the beds stained by the bodily fluids of other women was a deeply mortifying and stigmatising ordeal. In referring to menstrual blood as 'unclean' Noor was clearly making a reference to Muslim attitudes, but one that is by no means universally shared by all ethnic cultures in this region (Appell, 1991; Davison and Sutlive, 1987). For Noor, however, being obliged to lie in the menstrual blood of other women was a deeply degrading and contemptuous practice in the dehumanising process of turning individuals into patients.

My early interviews with patients on the acute wards involved soliciting questions concerning what constituted a 'typical day' on the ward, in due accordance with Spradley's (1979) formula of probing for comparisons and dissimilarities. The question was treated with as much interest by my participants as was the dawning of each new day for them in institutional care.

I learned through narrative and personal experience that on Female Ward 1 and Male Ward 1 the day started before dawn, from 5.00 am onwards there was movement on the wards and some patients would already be sleepily showering and getting dressed. The majority however, remained slumbering through this activity until they were obliged to rise to take their first daily dose of medication a short while later; they might then return to bed until rallied again for breakfast, following which some would inevitably attempt to sleep again. The routine revolved around the taking of medications, meal times, chores and sleep, and this set the monotonous tempo for the coming day, one that would have been highly familiar to past generations of psychiatric inmates across time and place.

For Jacob, a highly articulate, socially isolated, multiply admitted Chinese man in his early thirties, the most important question revolved around which medical assistant would be on duty that day. Those who had the ability to break the inertia of life on the ward were highly valued in comparison with those who are content with the soporific, unregulated passing of time.

Zulhan (MA) is the only one who makes a real difference for me, and he's the only one who has been trained ... in Singapore for 1 year. He sets tasks, which may look simple from the outside. We wake up early, take medicines and make our beds very nicely. His standard is very high. We shift tables, cut grass, wash and dry the dishes, do the laundry. And we do other things, like role play - like a father and his son or daughter passing by the shops and the child is ... not behaving. Zulhan sets up the scene and the things he wants to see happening. Sometimes we play netball or run round the compound. With the other MAs time passes monotonously. They do their tasks but do not organise patients into any activity particularly - very boring. Other MAs have a very low expectation of the patients and a rather limited view of their duties. Some MAs seem more like a policeman or a detective when he gets angry.

Jacob interpreted the organised routine set by the energetic, motivated Zulhan as indicative of his interest in the patients, and furthermore, his respect for their potential. The lack of stimulation provided by other members of staff was seen as a form of neglect, rather than liberalism and quite insulting in the practical implication that psychiatric patients are incorrigibly apathetic, and that their main requirements are simply met through tending to their animal needs and pacification, as provided by medication.

Responses to the same question posed on Female Ward 1 were rather different; the tedium of life on the wards was a noted feature, and a more or less expected one. More animation was expressed on the topic of food, which was usually listed as one of the main aggravations of ward life typified in the following quote from one woman: 'It is hard for me. I have no money! The food here is no good! Cannot go out!'

Aini was a witty, eloquent, popular Malay woman in early middle age and, like Jacob, had much experience of the hospital over the years. Despite all the indignities of ward life Aini exuded confidence and self-command, and was suitably disenchanted and scathing in her appraisal of life on the ward compared to life at home.

Aini:	The good and brilliant place for people is home. This is not a place for people, for animals!
Researcher:	In what way is this place for animals?
Aini:	The people (other patients) are very angry ... snatching at food like savages. ...The food is bad!'

Mealtimes, therefore, were an important theme in the narratives of patients, the three early mealtimes and two snacks broke the monotony and measured the time of a 'typical day'. Teo, a much hardened, veteran patient on Male Ward 1, ruefully commented that so far as he was concerned meals were about the only thing to look forward to. As Aini observed however, the food on the public wards was unpalatable and unvaried and seemed to be the worst of institutional cooking, grumbled over by Chinese patients occasionally, for being *halal* to boot, regardless of the preponderance of Chinese patients at the hospital (Ashencaen Crabtree, 2001).

A quotidian diet consisting of mounds of steamed rice, stewed vegetables and a small helping of protein - meat, fish or eggs formed the basis for meals. Food arrived in large tureens from the hospital kitchens and was slopped into bowls or army-style tray containers to be eaten in rapid privacy by patients. Meals were not used as a time for socialising, but on the contrary, privacy and solitude were emphasised more at these times than at other times of the day, as the following extract from field notes conveys.

Field notes: Male Ward 1.

Lunchtime begins at 11.20 am. A member of staff and Boon Chieng (a patient) serve out the food, which today is minced beef stew with cubed potatoes in it, steamed rice and mixed bean sprouts and greens. Tepid coffee to drink. The staff take plates of the food to those in the locked section. Open ward patients carry food to the table or sit on the veranda floor to eat. Food is a solitary experience, it would seem, with little talking going on but great concentration on the food, heads bowed over bowls or bowls lifted up to faces. In the locked section I notice that to gain privacy everyone sits with their backs to the bars facing the veranda - a curious sight of rows of backs is seen. Within 10-15 minutes the meal is over and clearing up by patients begin. Plastic dishes are stacked up in a huge bowl on the floor and hosed down by squatting patients.

For male patients at liberty to leave Male Ward 1, poor food could be supplemented by a visit to the canteen situated just inside the hospital's front gates, and for a fee of money or cigarettes were brought back to men confined on the wards. The canteen was nominally for the staff but patients were known to use it, as did the general public, particularly soldiers from the nearby barracks. It was predominantly patronised by men, albeit of very diverse status. Women patients were rarely able to use its facilities due to the tighter restrictions placed on their movements, although evidently some attempted to get nurses to buy extra food for them, judging from this rather bizarre and deeply mistrustful account from embittered, newly admitted Maslia on Female Ward 1. Although her claims could not be verified by me, her complaints could be construed as a counterattack on the context of marginalisation in which she struggled to survive (Lemert, 1993b).

> *But the nurse here is not honest. They (the nurses) simply cook the food and it's not tasty and well-cooked. Also, sometimes patients will ask nurses to buy food for them and the nurse lie to the patients saying that they bought the food for them, but actually the nurse cooked it themselves and sell it to the patients who wanted to eat those food. Besides, if there are additional food in the ward, the nurses didn't give it to the patients but instead, they eat it themselves.*

If gender played its part in the nutrition of patients, so too did class in relation to financial resources, whereby those in the private wards received a much improved diet, higher in protein, varied, well cooked and well presented. Although I have no evidence that women patients occupying a lower social class were subject to overt distinctions in relation to diet, the system ensured that their access to a superior level of nourishment, as enjoyed by other categories of patients, was effectively denied or made highly problematic.

At Hospital Tranquillity, patients were allocated a hospital uniform, although exceptions to this could be seen on both acute wards. Occasionally patients might be seen wearing a curious assortment of various-sized clothing, which were items of communal property left behind by previous patients and these were worn more in the spirit of 'dressing-up', and as such were tolerated by staff. Normally, however, the vast majority of patients wore the ubiquitous uniform, and this procedure took on overtones of ritualised initiation, or indeed 'mortification', upon entry to the wards (Goffman, 1991).

As such, the implications behind the wearing of a uniform formed a recurrent theme and was one that was almost exclusively discussed by women patients. Here an extract from field notes gives an illustration of the ritualistic and punitive socialisation into ward conventions of a Dayak woman from a remote area of Sarawak, in an illuminating modern-day evocation of prudish missionary zeal struggling to reform rebellious half-naked natives.

Field Notes: Female Ward 1.

The nurses are engaged in an exasperating attempt to educate a new patient in the locked ward into the niceties of behaviour. This patient apparently comes from a remote rural location, the staff say, and I have the impression that this is used as a way of explaining her unorthodox behaviour. She appears to be a wizened, diminutive woman, maybe only in her late forties to mid-fifties, who appears to be disabled, with a malformed hip, resulting in a curious staggering, stooping gait as she drags herself angrily around the locked section.

Now they are trying to get her to wear a hospital *baju* (jacket) as well as the regulation baggy shorts, which are so large on her small frame that she has pulled them right up to cover her chest. This, at least, for the nurses is a step in the right direction, as up till now she insisted on being bare-breasted, which is a normal state of dress in her traditional Dayak *kampung*. This is very much disapproved of by the nurses, Malay, Dayak and Chinese. The nurses make it clear to me that her obstinate nudity is a clear indication of her generally benighted, backward state; and every attempt is made to cajole her or demand that she conforms to the conventions of wearing the hospital uniform. I am given to understand that until she starts to behave in a 'reasonable' fashion, in other words compliant to ward rules and docile in manner, she will remain on the locked ward.

The whole issue of uniforms at Hospital Tranquillity is of course one of the more notorious features of life in psychiatric hospitals. The historical connection with the UK, that both informed and transformed health care in Malaysia over a relatively long period of colonial influence, encourages parallels to be drawn between asylum care across the two nations. Clark's dismal description of the impersonal allocation of communal, hospital clothing at Fulbourn Hospital in the England of the 1930s and 1940s is strongly reminiscent of Tranquillity today.

All clothing belonged to the hospital. It was regularly gathered and dispatched to the hospital laundry and there boiled. There was no individual clothing, not even underwear. In some women's wards a basketful of knickers would be dumped on the floor and the women would then scramble to get into something that might fit. The apathetic invariably ended up with clothes that did not fit .... All this was seen as an indication of their mental disorder and self-neglect (Clark, 1996: 55).

At Tranquillity patients were issued with robust and androgynous outfits consisting of anonymous and shapeless jackets and baggy culottes with the hospital initials printed on the breast pocket. A token nod at gender differences could be seen in the colour of uniforms rather than the shape, with most male patients dressed in grey or green, and most women in faded red gingham or navy blue (although a more unisex, drab green uniform is increasingly prevalent). These durable uniforms fulfilled two roles: being subjected to communal wear and laundering, they had a practical necessity and, as Gittins (1998) and Goffman point out, they acted as a symbol of a more profound personal dispossession (Goffman, 1991: 28).

> The uniformity and harshness of hospital clothing constantly reminded patients of their loss of status, freedom and identity (Gittins, 1998: 135).

Although the staff seemed largely oblivious to the attitudes patients had towards wearing the uniform, at least amongst some women respondents, the implications of the uniform were fully understood and accordingly deeply resented.

Field notes: Female Ward 1.

Aini joins us at this point, sits down and we proceed to talk about clothing. Full of boyish ardour and enthusiasm, Soo Mei, soon to be discharged, isn't wearing a uniform as usual but instead looks clean and dapper in her own tailored shorts and sports shirt. Aini says of course the patients here don't want to wear the uniform. I decide to draw her out on the subject.

Researcher:	So how do you feel about wearing a uniform Aini?
Aini:	Very depressive. Very bad feeling. You see the label here – 'Mental X'. People know you are mental.
Soo Mei:	(inquiringly) Mental? Something wrong?
Aini:	Yes, something wrong in the mind. People scared of you. When they know what you are wearing, they are scared of you.
Soo Mei:	And if you don't want to wear it they lock you up.
Aini:	[Looking at Soo Mei's outfit thoughtfully] You are not mental.
Soo Mei:	But if I am not mental why I here, *bodoh* (stupid)? [general laughter].

Aini:	[Referring to Soo Mei's clothing still] ... No one will suspect anything.
Soo Mei:	I getting slowly and slowly well ....
Aini:	(Disagreeing) Mentally retarded.
Soo Mei:	Yes, and she [pointing to me] is mentally retarded too [more laughter].

On another day, I talked to eloquent Aini again about uniforms, a subject she feels strongly about.

Aini:	When we go home we change clothes ... (the uniform) showing we are mentally retarded people ... not good, badly, desperate! Wearing a label 'XX' (Hospital Tranquillity) - all the people know who we are.

As Aini rightly pointed out, the uniform was a deeply stigmatising label making a clear public statement of the wearer's deviant status in society. While men were hardly better dressed they tended to present an indifferent attitude to the situation, but women seemed to find this a more painful issue. Women in Malaysia, as in the West, are expected to look attractive and attempt to 'make the best' of themselves. Women patients, especially in contrast with the spruce nurses, appeared all the more conspicuously dowdy therefore in their unbecoming uniforms. This was clearly a situation that others were aware of, as demonstrated by one male patient who said to me confidingly, 'but the women they look so ... *awful*. All their prettiness gone.' Yet in England back in 1932 the champion of women psychiatric patients, the reformer Dame Ellen Pinsent, was already caustically commenting on the uniforms in common use saying, 'Only advanced dementia would reconcile the average woman to the type of garment still worn in some hospitals' (Jones, 1993: 137). Uniform therefore served to desexualise modern-day Malaysian women patients, which symbolised a further fall in status, as an unkempt appearance shared by both sexes did not otherwise serve to level the unequal playing field between the position of men and women patients.

As a powerful visual symbol, the uniform is a more significant loss of status than simply being on the ward. On one occasion during a discussion about uniforms, Aini suddenly turned to Soo Mei and questioned her status as a patient due to her sporty 'civilian' attire: was she in fact really a patient? Soo Mei reasoned the matter out and asked rhetorically why on earth anyone, other than a member of staff, would voluntarily remain on the ward. That to do so was clearly an indication of mental illness, and so therefore, that might also explain the anomaly of my presence too!

By this time most patients and particularly the women of Female Ward 1 had become familiar with my odd visitations and even stranger questions. Here, however, I had a clear indication that I had been to some extent embraced in a discourse that could rightly be seen as subversive. My position as the butt of the joke indicated that I had achieved a new stage in my relationship with them and had managed to step out of the role of absolute outsider in this mischievous and humorous reversal, where I was evidently labelled as the mad one. The bantering tone teasingly questioned my motives and my sanity; also hinting that further reassurance was needed by me to establish why I had chosen to be amongst them. In particular it provided a deep insight into the perceptions of my participants in which questions were raised about the endless ambiguity of defining what *is* madness - a question often raised in sociologies of deviance (Rosenhan, 1993). For Aini and Soo Mei, in turn, there were a lot of people in the hospital who seemed to be mad but were not, and alternatively a lot who were not seen to be, but probably were, myself included.

The issue of power, such as that carried by the weight of labelling and that held by staff over patients, is one that recurred as a theme throughout fieldwork. Friendship among patients could mitigate the impact of highly unequal power differentials, and as such, social networks across patient groups were of great importance. The exercise of power among patients was played out as overtly as between that of staff and patients, where many sought to cultivate the patronage of individuals regarded as particularly high ranking within the patient hierarchy. The next chapter focuses upon these social dynamics among patient groups, and particularly the rise of a cadre of a patient elite.

Note

1   *Bejalai* refers to the Iban male's right to rove in search of adventure or employment for months and years on end (Mashman, 1991: 261). Iban women are in turn expected to remain at home to ensure the survival of the family and its fortunes.

5
Ward relationships:
Power and reciprocation

In the closed confines of the ward environment, the hierarchical structure inevitably looms large for patients in relation not only to staff, but also to their peers. Ward life, as Goffman points out, is the definitive example of the 'total institution' in which all functions of life are carried out within the institutional setting and according to its definitions, requirements and mandates (Goffman, 1991: 11). As such, the ward tends to magnify peer relationships as inescapable webs of influence that encompass and dominate the social existence of patients to a large degree. The complexities of interactions at ward level in this study, and which equally enmeshed the researcher, could be identified as a number of different relational patterns that were thrown into sharp relief by the otherwise depersonalised and regimented life to which patients were expected to conform.

Unfortunately, comparisons are not always easy to draw between the conditions of life in modern institutions compared to historical ones. As Roy Porter (2006) argues the voices of the mad are largely missing from the accounts of insanity in asylum care, compared to the weight of medical accounts, owing largely to the belief that their utterances were not considered worth recording. Therefore, and in relation to the themes covered in this chapter, it is hard to contextualise historically the quality of relationships in custodial settings, particularly eighteenth-century Georgian 'madhouses', the subject of Porter's thesis, many of which were notorious, although some frankly luxurious. These Georgian units typically held small numbers of fee-paying inmates who were frequently sent home within six months (Porter, 2006). By contrast the large Victorian asylums may well have been more likely to offer conditions where long term relationships could more easily be developed between patient peers and across patient-staff hierarchies, particularly as many of these interactions are formed through the discipline of the ward routine and the labour generated by it, as examples from Tranquillity duly indicate.

Reciprocal relationships

The notion of friendship amongst patients at Tranquillity provoked some interesting responses. First-admission patients were usually still in the painful process of adjustment, and other patients on the ward were often dismissed as being merely a motley collection of *orang gila* (mad people). As such, the implication was that they were of no direct consequence to anybody, and consequently this derogatory term could also be used by established patients in discrediting former friends.

For those patients, men and women, on the acute wards who had experienced multiple admissions, the ward, however, was more likely to represent a sociable environment where they might encounter a relatively high level of acceptance and camaraderie, in comparison to the isolation and rejection that often characterised life 'at home'. This patient 'sub-culture' appeared to acts as an important buffer between the self-esteem of the individual and the social rejection that the role of mental illness imposed upon them within their own communities (Barham and Hayward, 1996: 234).

Friends, for example, were a big issue for Dimbaud, who had been admitted more than twenty times over the last ten years, and confessed that he was lonely back at his Dayak longhouse. This was a significant issue considering the traditional close-knit nature of such communities (Mashman, 1987; Schmidt, 1964). Abang, who once lived in a Malay *kampung* (village), agreed, adding that his friends were those here in the hospital and that there was no one he could really call a friend outside of the hospital anymore.

> *My friends (in the hospital) very nice, very friendly. I don't have friends at home ... Been here for 4 to 5 years, but I do go back for home leave.about one week. I just gone back ... but this time I come back earlier, not really one week ... Last time (undefined past) I have friends but now they already working. They don't worry about me. If they work they don't care about me anymore. They did not find me to play hockey, football ....*

Due to the loss of common ground, relationships with 'normals' tend to deteriorate over time until connections between individuals and their communities are ultimately too attenuated to bridge gaps in erstwhile friendships (Estroff, 1984). Respondents were strongly aware of this situation and several indicated that they did not find this a welcome topic to discuss, and a deeper insight into loss of personal connections was therefore not easily obtainable.

Some people like Jacob on Male Ward 1 were particularly isolated, as he had no real friends on the ward, and seemingly none in the community either. The business of just getting along with others was seen as a very poor substitute for finding a close friend, something Jacob yearned for, but in this attempt he seemed doomed to frustration.

> *The majority of people on the ward are of low education – they haven't finished Form 3 (primary education). Only about 10% have the kind of education I have. It's impossible to make good friendships on the ward because people are so sick. and sometimes I haven't had a very good response when I've tried to ask them questions.*

Unfortunately, for Jacob, despite his obvious intelligence, he had little insight into the feelings of others and therefore the kinds of questions he asked were often inflammatory, such as 'do your family visit you?' This was a fascinating issue for Jacob in view of his stormy and alienated family relations, but a very tactless question to ask in a context where so many had been estranged from their families for years, with dire results for their future. As a result Jacob attempted to define his relationship with his favourite medical assistant, Zulhan, as a 'friendship' of sorts because of the lively and caring interactions he received from this particular professional. By the nature of things this could not be a 'symmetrical' relationship, as Estroff puts it, and the most basic condition for friendship could not be realised (1984: 250).

Friendships on the ward amongst patient peers clearly represented an important source of emotional support, but also acted as a necessary social lubricant in a congested communal space occupied by large numbers of diverse individuals. To this end casual friendships and general bonhomie were in fact the conditions necessary for survival on the wards and therefore cordial and reciprocal relations were by far the most prevalent types of relationship found amongst participants. These types of relationships, however, could also be viewed as temporary alliances rather than genuine friendships, and were quite often built on a brittle foundation of expediency and mutual benefit that could quite quickly turn to enmity.

I found Tuyah, a long-stay but still youthful Dayak patient on Female Ward 1, to be a mercurial character. A mixture of cheerful indifference verging on the callous, combined with grandiose pretensions to power, she was nearly always game for a long animated chat. Tuyah took a sanguine attitude to life pointing out that living under ward conditions a person is obliged to rub shoulders with all manner of individuals without the luxury of too much discrimination.

(This ward) holds all sorts of people. Many are very sick. They have no control over their bowels; they wander around, their eyeballs roll up; they shake or drop their heads down. Here are all kinds of people: Malay, Bidayuh, Iban, Melanau, Chinese.

Subsequently people like Tuyah were careful to ensure that arguments were kept to a minimum, and a general network of good relations was fostered with most people on the ward. The confined and claustrophobic universe that the ward represented meant that enmities could not be allowed to flourish unchecked. It was all the more important therefore to ensure that one had friends who could be relied on to share an odd cigarette or snack. In fact, *sharing* is what makes a friend, added Mariam, Tuyah's multiply admitted Malay chum.

Reciprocation amongst patients represented a common theme uniting them on all the wards I studied. A few members of staff interpreted sharing behaviour as being examples of an altruistic gesture, or as one nurse put it, 'patients are very generous to each other'. On the male wards a medical assistant observed that some patients had to be prevented from giving coveted items away. Based on interviews with patient participants of both sexes, however, it emerged that those who do not share risk exclusion from the vital network of mutual support. This raises the conditions of merely surviving on the wards to a higher level of comfort and enjoyment. Some patients like the aloof Tan Siew could afford to opt out of the reciprocal network due to private means, which, although relatively limited, nonetheless represented quite a sizable sum on Male Ward 1. Tan Siew was a rather dissolute middle-aged Chinese patient originally from Sibu, East Malaysia, who had a long history of admissions interspersed by periods of destitution. Thanks however to the pocket money forwarded by his otherwise absent family, he retained his independent status on the ward. Although his general reputation also held that he was untrustworthy, sly and manipulative, this did not seem to visibly trouble him, if indeed he was aware of his notoriety at all. Consequently, 'cadging' and sharing were not uppermost on his mind as it was for many of his fellow inmates. 'A cigarette' said Tan Siew, 'is like a wife': which in other words you do not share. Although evidently he could be generous with his cigarette butts when he chose, thus maintaining cordial if subservient relationships commensurate with his lofty but friendless status on the ward.

Through chats with Mariam and Tuyah, I learned that staff sometimes presented themselves as friends to the patients for reasons of their own, but since they did not share their belongings this was construed as just false camaraderie. Without it being explicitly said, the message is that this was of course also true of me. On at least three occasions I received gifts from individuals, one being from a nurse, while the other two were from women patients, who gave me respectively a tiny sachet of instant coffee and a much-used personal ornament. Unfortunately, as I did not understand the significance of these overtures at the time, I did not return these favours and therefore presumably I failed to create the necessary conditions for genuine friendship. Nonetheless, patients of both sexes saw me as a figure of some influence in the hospital, and often referred to me by the powerful title of 'doctor', either by mistake or through ingratiation.

Women and men quickly identified me as a probable source of help and I was subject to frequent petitioning by patients to exert myself on their behalf. In this way I found myself reluctantly placed in a role that conformed closely to that of the 'rescuer' as defined by Asher and Fine (1991: 202), a role of power in itself. As a 'rescuer' I was regularly asked to intervene on the behalf of patients to obtain a rapid discharge, or to provide them with money or other covetable items. Occasionally I was asked to find employment for patients once discharged, as exemplified by Linda's plea, 'Talk to the *towkay* (shop owner/boss) for me ... I don't think they want to employ people from here'. Now and again, I was even asked to employ a patient participant myself. Margot for example, asked me if I would consider taking her on as a personal servant, but without waiting for my answer responded despondently that no doubt I was looking for someone much younger and fitter that she was.

While I found these petitions and the assumptions that lay behind them extremely embarrassing, I was also aware of having been hoist by my own petard, in that evidently my colonial baggage had finally caught up with me despite any pretensions to the contrary, at least so far as patients were concerned. As a white person, even one whose appearance was made deliberately nondescript, I was perceived to be powerful, wealthy and privileged, and therefore easily able to grant favours and use my influence should I so wish.

Many long-serving patients could recall a time when the medical hierarchy at Tranquillity had been dominated by colonial powers, and therefore it was quite logical to identify me with these figures of authority. Margot's assumption that I was in the business of recruiting domestic staff was in this context a reasonable supposition, given that colonials would of course employ local staff in this way, and that it is likely that some ex-psychiatric patients might find employment through these routes. Field work implied that I was indebted to the participants involved and therefore, on a *quid pro quo* basis at least, the implication was that I was expected to return the favour. The uneven situation that I found myself in, whereby I was unable to reward participants in the tangible ways they suggested, resonated uncomfortably with Judith Stacey's point (1991) that the research encounter is essentially a one-sided, exploitative exercise. That said, such petitions actually underlined the inherently unequal status between myself and patient participants; to comply with them, had it been in my power to do so, would only have served to perpetuate these inequalities rather than rectify or even address them.

Finally, as a woman and one who had worked hard to forge good relationships with both women and men on the wards, it was not unreasonable for patients to assume that this indicated an inclination on my part to share tangible benefits with others less privileged. The assumption by women patients that I would be particularly empathic towards women was correct, and by some strange extension was at the basis of my relationship with *Miss* Hui Ling. This fragile-looking young patient on Male Ward 1 had at some point prior to admission adopted a fully-fledged transsexual identity that was maintained here in the face of staff ridicule and the obvious lack of suitable accessories and props. In fact, it seemed to me that confinement on a male ward strongly reinforced an exaggeratedly feminine identity, which was treated with a certain public chivalry by fellow patients; although whether this was exploited sexually in private remains unknown. Accordingly, Hui Ling frequently engaged me in conversation, bemoaning the horrors of being incarcerated in a ward full of coarse men, and which 'as a woman also', I could surely identify with her predicament and accordingly secure her release.

The 'sharing' of goods operates in at least two different ways, first as a way of securing friends and improving one's quality of life. Second, items can be used as a means of making a profit, usually through a system of barter and payment in kind, rather than through ready cash, although the latter was a feature of ward life as well.

Cigarettes, to reiterate, formed the primary goods in this informal marketplace of profiteering, with food and sweets seemingly taking a less prominent position, due perhaps as one nurse suggested to problems of access. For many patients, male and female, chronic and acute, the main activities revolved around smoking, which in common with other psychiatric institutions was rife at the hospital (Goffman, 1991). Staff accounts variously point out that cigarettes, as opposed to food, are easily obtainable from friendly, or perhaps somewhat intimidated, visitors to the hospital, and that smoking acts as a form of initiation for new patients, even those who are nonsmokers at the point of admission. One nurse put the prevalence of smoking down to 'boredom' and peer example. In addition, a long-serving nurse pointed out that in the past it was commonplace practice to hand cigarettes out to patients 'as an incentive for good behaviour'. Tobacco was typically used by staff in traditional psychiatric institutions in Britain in a similar manner: as a form of reward, and consequently as positive reinforcement for behaviour, as well as a means of punishing addicted patients through deprivation of their 'fix' (Rutherford, 2008).

Cigarettes, therefore, formed the main commodity in the market place, in which commercially made cigarettes were bulked out by the even cheaper homemade variety made of a toxic combination of the contents of cigarette butts wrapped around *atap* thatch made from palm fronds. If an opportunity occurred these were fairly discreetly hawked around male and female wards as an acceptable and affordable substitute for the real thing, when it could not be paid for, begged, borrowed or stolen.

Men appear to dominate as entrepreneurs, with only a tiny minority of women participating in these activities, such as the resourceful, independent Catherine on Female Ward 2. Culturally Malaysian women of most ethnic groups have always had a foothold in mercantile activities, and have not been excluded from producing and profiting in the marketplace (Davison and Sutlive, 1987; Karim, 1995; Padmini Selvaratnam, 2001). The low profile of women in marketing activities at Tranquillity, therefore, suggests that there were other causes at work to account for their exclusion, which is discordant with ethnic and gender expectations in this multicultural society.

Wily Mathew from Male Ward 2, a sinewy Dayak chronic patient of indeterminate age, was an excellent source of information on the activities of the opportunistic male dealer, and through extrapolation provided some good insights into the absence of women entrepreneurs. Considered fairly dependable by the staff, who could usually trust him to return to the ward in good time, he was usually given permission to go out on rambles round the hospital. Mathew in turn, however, often took advantage of the situation to go *jalan jalan*, or in other words strolled into town through the simple expedient of sneaking out of the hospital grounds.

Once free, Mathew made his regular rounds of the local cafes, visiting proprietors in order to scrounge whatever he could. He was usually successful in this venture, since to submit to his fairly modest demands was probably the easiest way to get rid of him. On his return to the hospital Mathew hawked his goods amongst inmates on the different wards, if necessary carrying out transactions through the barred grill gates, or alternatively confined his activities to his own ward for added social lubrication.

Fortunately, for Mathew he was first and foremost a male patient, and a harmless one at that, for while male patients could occasionally be seen in town, and were conspicuous as such by their hospital uniform, much greater vigilance was employed in the care of women patients. The access of women patients to the general hospital grounds was subject to much greater restriction and therefore women patients were practically never seen beyond the walls of the hospital. Restricted access to sources of supply, as well as the difficulties involved in accessing customers on other wards, effectively and heavily curtailed the activities of women dealers. Female patients were thereby relegated to the less profitable role of passive consumers of cigarettes, whilst due to the repercussions of trading restrictions, and other means of increasing personal revenue, they were more likely to be able to afford only the cheapest and most harmful type of cigarette available.

'Sharing' and profiteering carry with them the inherent danger of being involved in conflicts over possession and this was a main cause of fights on the ward. For as Tuyah and Mathew pointed out, there were characters on the ward who enjoyed victimising others and stealing their goods, because there was 'something wrong with their brains'. While 'old hands' were aware of these hazards and took steps to avoid unpleasant encounters, for newcomers, such as Elvis, a homesick, bewildered Bidayuh sixteen-year-old, enduring his first incarceration at the hospital, these fights were a frightening event.

Field notes. Male Ward 1.

Elvis makes a violent, throat-grasping gesture as he describes the kind of fights, which break out amongst patients. Quarrels break out over small things, such cigarettes, bullying or bragging. But says Elvis, 'the worst thing is that they go on until they are stopped – or *kill* someone'.

Elvis's notion that murder and mayhem are a feature of ward life was in fact based more on fantasy than reality. As such, this represented the extreme anxiety he felt at being diagnosed as mentally ill and being misplaced in a Bedlam of unpredictable violence. For Elvis, insanity *was* precisely this kind of alarming, immoderate behaviour, to which he was currently struggling to attach meaning and motive. Although Elvis's fear of murder was an exaggerated one, the fear of being involved in a violent episode is a completely understandable one in view of what the Sainsbury Centre for Mental Health (1998: 5) call the 'small but serious risk of violence' on psychiatric wards . Just as fights and violence feature on the psychiatric ward in Britain, at Tranquillity this was an ever present, if not necessarily, a highly hazardous situation for most patients on the wards.

Dominant relationships

Acts of violence on the ward might break out as seemingly spontaneous aggression that was usually swiftly broken up by ward staff. Violence by patients was also used covertly as a means of ensuring discipline on the wards, while staff assaults were an infrequent, but by no means unknown event, according to the discreet hint given to me by one house doctor. In this case, aggression by patients towards patients did not conform to the more commonplace strife that was subject to staff control. Instead, staff appeared to collude in aggressive conduct that was demonstrated by individuals, who despite being patients themselves, were placed in a position of power over their peers:

> We had already learned that those wearing striped clothing were prisoners like us… This made it all the more difficult to understand why they treated us so viciously… (Kielar, 1982: 6).

A good deal of fieldwork elapsed before I began to differentiate the few acts of violence I witnessed into type, nature, motive and most importantly, consequence. Eventually I began to appreciate more fully the dominant role played by several patients on both the acute and chronic wards. This cadre of powerful individuals among the patients were a heterogeneous mix, but the one aspect they had in common was that they appeared to stand distinct from the ward mass and often carried both influence and the bearing of insignia of higher standing, in terms of dress or privilege. For want of a better expression, I adopted the term 'prominent', as used by Primo Levi, in writing of his Auschwitz experience, to describe those prisoners raised above the ordinary lot (Levi, 1979: 96). I use the term advisedly as I certainly do not want to imply that conditions at Hospital Tranquillity are in any way comparable to life in a Lager. Nonetheless, it seems to me that the general role of control of peers by an appointed elite amongst the patient corps is central to the phenomenon, as I understand it, enacted on the ward, and is in some ways analogous to the 'boss boy' role of the African foreman in colonial Southern Rhodesia (Jackson, 2005: 82)

If the drowned have no story, and single and broad is the path to perdition, the paths to salvation are many, difficult and improbable (Levi, 1990: 96).

To generalise then, the ward *prominent* occupied a privileged position in relation to other members on the ward, and this position was endorsed through action or omission to act by the real authorities on the ward, the staff. Not all wards appeared to have an obvious coterie of *prominents*, yet this was noticeable on many. Evidently, this was a useful role on the ward, as it was not uncommon to find individuals like these helping out with all manner of tasks, rarely menial, but more often supervisory, managerial and disciplinary in some fashion or another. Some *prominents* were fairly innocuous individuals and were rarely if ever involved in bullying others, at least physically. Others, and these of both sexes, could be seen to be outright bullies and openly aggressive in their behaviour towards others. On Female Ward 2 force was used to maintain the authority of Martha, a sullen and menacing woman, who had few words to spare for anybody, but plenty of spirit to punish perceived transgression. Martha was a capable individual on a ward characterised by a majority of disabled individuals. She frequently acted literally as 'door-keeper', keeping a close eye on those who wanted to enter and leave the ward, and was often privileged with locking and unlocking the gate herself, after a dour scrutiny of visitors, such as myself, who wished to enter or leave. Personally, I found Martha an unpleasant and unpredictable individual, with overtly bullying habits gratuitously inflicted seemingly for the sheer pleasure of maintaining her fearsome reputation, as the following brief example illustrates.

Field notes. Female Ward 2

Martha Chung has a permanently sullen expression. Her name is down on several rotas for cleaning floors, making beds etc. Obviously she is seen as one of the most capable patients but she also has a very unpleasant side. I see her pass by the locked ward containing a very confused Chinese patient and poke her in the face with a fist (pulling back so that it is less than a punch) but getting no real reaction Martha then slaps her in the face and threatens her with a scowl and a fist before moving off in her independent swaggering gait.

Violence was far from unknown on this ward, despite the general stereotypic belief at Tranquillity that violence and aggression are not typical characteristics of women. This was demonstrated by the fact that there are no resources for violent female offenders at Tranquillity, although there were such people here, while women are generally regarded by staff as more 'compliant' and easier to manage than men (Orme, 1994). Aggression on Female Ward 2 was usually punished with a spell on the locked section, however, I never saw Martha incarcerated in this fashion, much as she might deserve to be in all fairness. Additionally, although Martha had comparatively menial tasks to do on the ward, yet in a ward where so few were as capable as she, her chores marked her out as one of superior abilities. Martha's cooperation in this respect rewarded her with more important tasks and a privileged status, free from much interference by the ward staff.

Catherine was something of an enigma on Female Ward 2. First of all, it was not easy to calculate her real age, for although Catherine had the gait, as well as the personal wardrobe of a young woman, any freshness she may have held had long since turned stale leaving her ageless but without youth. Irrespective of this, Catherine as a veteran patient had become a successful entrepreneur who had risen in rapidly in the ranks achieving the status of a *prominent*. In common with Martha, Catherine exercised a lot of power but this was strictly confined to the pursuit of her own ends, these being predominantly connected to personal comfort and autonomy. Because Catherine was considered to be a very competent individual, at one point it was hoped that she would be able to thrive in NGO-run supported accommodation. This, however, was not a successful placement and Catherine was returned to the custodial care of the hospital, as it was found that she refused to develop the necessary independent living skills. Instead Catherine seemed to prefer to use a variety of unpleasant forms of coercion, including physical intimidation, to force other residents to support her.

On the ward, Catherine continued to exploit others through similar tactics and seemed quite content to be back in the hospital environment, being one of the few women permitted to leave the ward more or less as she pleased. This enabled her 'businesses' to flourish, and in addition she enjoyed the support and protection of her well-connected and involved family. Her general appearance was strikingly fashionable in comparison with her peers on the ward and she exuded an air of complacent guile. Catherine's power apparently lay in her ability to shirk chores and delegate these to others, leaving her free to enjoy an almost unequalled level of freedom and leisure amongst women patients, leaving open the question of how staff might be duly compensated for bestowing these valuable privileges.

On Female Ward 1, Tuyah was also engaged in seeking prominence. Her approach was to make use of her wide experience of the malign supernatural. Tuyah told me with some relish that she had been the victim of an *orang buat* (a witch or sorcerer) since her adolescence. During this prolonged possession she has been multiply raped by an *hantu* (a spirit being or incubus) and miniaturised animals, including a crocodile, were seen to emerge from her vagina (I assume this latter to have a sexual as well as cultural reference). Additionally, Tuyah's arms and legs were covered with a multitude of old and half-healed scars that look self-inflicted. Tuyah, however, had managed to acquire some status on the ward, although not as much as she would have liked, and was confident to the point of egomania at times. She announced herself to be a fully fledged *dukun*: a shamanistic healer of some consequence, able to detect and cure illness as well as communicate with the spirit world (Winzeler, 1995: 115).

> The shaman's role… is one of curing sick people using a range of supernatural techniques. Shamans are drawn into this role because of an experience considered by them to be an illness, an affliction, and a victimization by a spirit-being (Bernstein, 1993: 171).

To claim to be a *dukun*, a *manang* or *bomoh* carries important connotations for patients at Tranquillity, in a cultural context where so many patients have sought help at one time or another from traditional healers, and whose care is seen to be at least parallel to, if not equally as good as that of psychiatry (Loustaunau and Sobo, 1997; Razali, 1997).

Although tormented by her symptoms, which included excruciating headaches, bulging eyeballs, disorientation and fainting fits, Tuyah did not regard this as excluding her from the role of a *dukun* by virtue of her suffering or her sex, in fact quite the opposite applied. Illness and affliction are recognised amongst ethnic groups in Borneo to be one of the more obvious signs of a spiritual vocation that may be visited upon women, as well as men (Rousseau, 1993). The victimisation by spirits, often through highly sexualised overtures or other forms of attack, is a further indication of this calling, and it is far wiser to embrace this fate, rather than ignore or reject it (Bernstein, 1993). The suffering of the shaman initiate is not a minor inconvenience easily ignored but is intense and demanding.

> Knowledge comes to him (the shaman) during events of tremendous feeling – pain, ecstasy, and seizures, illness and trauma, at times self-inflicted…. In trances or in other altered states brought about by self-inflicted suffering, the shaman experiences 'torture', 'being cut to pieces', which lead to death and resurrection. (Romanucci-Ross, 1997b: 216).

While staff attributed a catalogue of distressing symptoms to mental illness, Tuyah knew that these were clear manifestations and indications of her spiritual calling. Although Tuyah's suffering was extravagant, and her descriptions of them most vivid, these signs of a greater destiny were to be flaunted amongst fellow patients, rather than denied or played down.

On Male Ward 1, Boon Chieng held a position that combined aspects of these seemingly polarised positions. Like Catherine, Boon Chieng was a man who stood aside from most patient interactions, and in comparison with the average patient had an agreeable appearance, being well dressed and urbane with a soldierly briskness to his movements. In comparison to Martha, he was a responsible and dependable supervisor of others and had specialised in the allocation of meals. His duties also encompassed access to the keys of the locked section, distribution of patient uniforms and bedding, as well as assisting in administering medication to others under the supervision of a member of staff. Fortunately, unlike Martha, Boon Chieng was a non-violent individual who managed to enforce his authority through other means, and probably those directly connected to his duties.

Having observed Boon Chieng for some time I was rather taken aback to hear a litany of very bizarre outpourings from him in a private interview situation. For Boon Chieng seemed totally preoccupied with the literal fear of being poisoned, and roundly accused relatives and ward staff of persistently trying to kill him. This then was the reason for his chosen and favourite duty of food attendant: he could keep a close eye on proceedings as a means of self-protection. With the status that this situation had brought about, seemingly Boon Chieng had gone on to consolidate his position of power by taking on still greater responsibility.

Boon Chieng's official diagnosis labelled him a paranoid schizophrenic and his obsessions certainly seemed to confirm this. Fortunately, however, as in Tuyah's case, his mental illness had not proved to be a handicap to him on the ward but rather the reverse: in that in many ways this had enabled Boon Chieng to make the most of available opportunities in achieving a high level of rank. For ward staff the outward appearance of 'mental stability' is a prerequisite for any credibility, and Boon Chieng's conduct demonstrated this stability, even though staff were fully aware of his innermost paranoia.

Like Boon Chieng, Jani the *prominent* ward entrepreneur on Male Ward 2, did not need to assert his position through physical aggression. Although he could boast of a burly, well-fed physique that would easily overpower most challengers, ferocity was not Jani's style. Instead, an air of single-minded self-preservation, rather than a bully's intimidation, marked him out from the crowd. Like Catherine on Female Ward 2 he had a 'business' that he attended to, which took him out of the ward regularly - staff turning a blind eye to these nefarious excursions. On his return a hopeful retinue of patients formed around him in the hope of cadging a cigarette that he might condescendingly pass over, as evidently most of his 'business' took place on other, probably more profitable, wards. Jani was clearly well linked into the underground system of procurement of coveted items and probably this, as well as his undeniable sense of himself and general coping ability, had helped him to attain this comfortable position.

Not all who would assume the position of *prominent* are accepted as such, despite attempts to emulate the appropriate behaviour. On Male Ward 1 Alias, an inarticulate Malay youth, showed many of the traits found in the successful *prominent*, but lacked the ability to attain the position. Alias resorted to standard tactics to elevate himself, such as attempting to undertake responsible jobs, as well as doing his best to physically threaten other patients.

Field notes. Male Ward 1.

On the open ward Alias is up to his odd antics. With a permanent and somewhat menacing scowl he glowers at me [I pretend not to be looking at him]; he unplugs the operating lights and fan; he prods at a plastic bowl under the nursing station and moves it a few millimetres with his foot; he picks up a bundle of folded towels and with precise violence bangs them down again on to the same spot; he picks up the remote control of the television and puts it away in a drawer. Then wanders off and shouts something at the patients on the locked ward, who ignore him.

Researcher: [to MA] He seems busy helping tidy up the place.
MA: No, he is looking for something … [moves off]

The fact is Alias isn't looking for anything but is going through the ritual of acting like a medical assistant: organising, inspecting and maintaining order amongst the patients. But the medical assistant denies this and does not see what is being enacted. Later I see him out of his old hospital uniform and wearing a lurid, flamboyant outfit but ill-fitting and improperly fastened.

Unfortunately for Alias and his ambitions, his behaviour was very unpredictable in that he often behaved like a buffoon and cavorted playfully with patients when he chose. His whimsical behaviour on the other hand often caused him to overstep his mark as a bully to no good purpose, or alternatively he would go too far in the aping of ward staff. In fact, despite how totally conditioned Alias was by the ward system, he was not a candidate for any real authority as staff could not exploit him adequately as an extra and dependable pair of hands, for he was seen to be incompetent due to Down's Syndrome, his limited comprehension and generally erratic behaviour.

Gaining status through these various routes is usually a fairly long-term strategy and therefore prominent individuals were almost exclusively found among long-stay patients, who had a vested interest in achieving the best possible place in the 'pecking order'. This approximates with Goffman's description of how established patients move on to make 'secondary adjustments', in which a partial or total acceptance of the realities of the alternative world of the asylum has been made (Goffman, 1991: 182). Likewise, at Tranquillity occasionally a particularly charismatic and assertive first-admission patient might attempt to gain a higher position in the ranking order. Usually, however, newly admitted patients were more likely to be overwhelmed by the need to make a rapid adjustment to the routines and rituals of the ward, and did not therefore represent a real threat to the established *prominents*.

In consequence, long-stay patients and staff were well known to each other and this familiarity did at times breed if not contempt amongst patients, a willingness to push the boundaries of authority as far as they could. While elitism amongst patients on the ward could be very useful, the problem for ward staff lay in maintaining the demarcation between their rank and that of the *prominent*, as *just* another patient. This resulted in a certain tension at times, whereby a *prominent* could be temporarily punished or even permanently demoted for stepping out of line by being reduced to the ranks. As an insolent and 'pushy' individual (in relation to staff) Tuyah spent a good deal of time in the locked ward. Likewise, garrulous Frankie on *Bunga Raya* Ward lost a coveted long-term position of rank that he worked hard for after arguing with the staff over the publicly acknowledged extent of his powers.

Conferring rank and privilege amongst select patients could therefore be seen to a useful strategy for relieving workloads for staff. This is also a highly effective means of control through the sowing of a divisive seed amongst patients, where the person most likely to be in a position to draw attention to subversive patient behaviour was the *prominent*, rather than the staff.

We are aware that this is very distant from the picture that is usually given of the oppressed who unite, if not in resistance, at least in suffering. (Levi, 1979: 97).

Not surprisingly therefore, to maintain privilege it was important that *prominents* upheld the rules of the ward and valued the ethos of the system, if not totally, at least sufficiently to maintain prestige and position as demotion was by no means unknown. Such a situation was liable to lead to rivalry amongst patients and acrimony, creating a necessity to rule by tyranny, as exemplified by Martha's behaviour; or by influence and beneficence, as exemplified by Tuyah's approach. In any event, the repercussions of privilege were unlikely to lead to the relinquishment of power by individual *prominents* in view of the advantages offered by the system.

Familial relationships and patient labour

Asylums, as a general rule, have utilised the labour of patients to maintain the institution, sometimes attempting to generate a financial return on institutional care through the unpaid or poorly paid labour of patients. A female patient's accounts from a nineteenth century asylum in America, for instance, briefly describes how degraded inmates were used as servants by staff and were required to accustom themselves to performing 'nearly all the drudgery' (Geller and Harris, 1994: 54). Therefore as Black (1988), and in addition Barham (1992), point out that psychiatric hospitals have long regarded patient labour as an essential commodity, and in this respect Tranquillity was no different. By and large, however, the work undertaken by patients was divided into two general types, of which ward chores might be supervised by *prominents*. This stood in accordance with one of the major roles undertaken by *prominents*, which in the context of the Lager is to assist in the exploitation of fellow inmates through their labour. Other forms of labour at Tranquillity were reframed as 'therapeutic' and managed by staff, thus camouflaging any vested interest the hospital may have in patient labour, as discussed further in the final section of this chapter.

A causal link between labour and a further type of relationship amongst patients existed that I identified as *familial* relationships, and these were adopted on wards as a specific cultural response to the social situation, as well as being a mode of interaction that operated to the advantage of ward staff. On most wards at Tranquillity it was not difficult to find examples of pseudo-family relationships, such as that on Male Ward 1 where frightened teenagers sought out the protection of older males as paternal figures. Similarly on Male Ward 3 a well-known patient senior in age, experience and ability 'fathered' many of his younger peers, and similar parental examples could be found on the female wards. As such, it is not suggested that these types of relationships were exclusive to Hospital Tranquillity, and indeed are no doubt replicated in some form or other on most psychiatric wards globally.

In Malaysia, however, the development of 'familial' types of relationships represent a specific cultural strategy for creating connections of rapport amongst non-related individuals, as described by Wazir Jahan Karim:

> In Malaysia and Indonesia a manifestation of this is the metaphorical naming (through terms of address) of people beyond the local grouping by kinships terms, as if to recreate the intimacy and familiarity of consanguinal and affinal ties in local groupings in other spheres of life. Everywhere patron-client and employer-employee relations in economic and political affairs are neutralised by terms like *pa'cik* (uncle) and *ma'cik* (aunty) in Malaysia. (Karim, 1995: 37).

Indeed so strong can these 'affinal' ties become that some members of staff develop very close 'familial response' to patients in their care. On Male Ward 3 a medical assistant described how a patient was reunited with his community after several years, and was then discharged home, only to be rapidly readmitted following difficulties in adjustment. 'He wanted to come back here - this is his home, and *we* are like his family' was the emotive explanation given. Although these types of relationships had an emotional role to play, on the chronic wards, and particularly the female chronic wards, familial relationships were premised upon labour and, as such, were encouraged by staff.

Field notes. Female Ward 2.

Patients are busy caring for others. This seems to be an important role for many patients - I see several helping older, incapacitated ones on the commode; taking them to the bathroom; changing their clothes. An older woman start to undress a diminutive, youthful figure that lies hopelessly curled up. Her legs have to be rearranged before the shorts can be removed, underneath she wears no underwear. She is half carried, half dragged by the older woman and a nurse to the bathroom. This is the severely disabled and probably brain-damaged young patient I have seen in the past. It is hard to guess her age but maybe in her early 20s. Later I see her slumped in a chair. Her face looks smooth, blank and expressionless.

The nurse tells me that this help is regarded as therapy; another says that originally the ward was so understaffed that patients had to help each other, now it has become a valuable feature of this ward. For instance, I am told, one patient regards an older one as a mother figure who cares for her almost totally, and the younger one describes herself as her *anak* (child).

The chronic wards held a comparatively large number of patients who were unable to care for themselves due to their mental and physical disabilities, and these people were therefore dependent on basic nursing skills. While the female staff were engaged in undertaking nursing tasks, these fundamentally incapacitated individuals were cared for by other patients, in a sort of informal 'twinning' programme. Commonly, more able women were expected to care for others, assisting them in washing, dressing, toileting and feeding activities on a daily basis. This was achieved through the forging of personal relationships between patients that was encouraged by staff, who used filial and parental terms to describe such bonding.

This situation is not unique to Hospital Tranquillity, however, but conforms closely to Ong's description of how Malay female factory workers are controlled through the use of pseudo-family roles and the associated ties of obligation. In the case of factory workers senior male staff consciously adopt the authority of the paterfamilias over subservient 'daughter' workers (Ong, 1995). Equally, in the hospital setting staff evidently benefited enormously from the caring relief provided by patients. It could nonetheless be argued that these nurturing alliances between patients could well have been extremely valuable to long-stay adults, who were otherwise barred from developing intimate relationships in society. The nurturing role is of course associated primarily with women stereotypically, and while it is true that this could be found on the male wards, it was far less commonplace. Another aspect of the heavy burden of care provided by female patients was that these chronic wards held a larger number of incapacitated patients than the male chronic wards, although ages and duration of stay were similar. This tended to suggest that incapacitated male patients were less likely to be cared for in the same way as female counterparts. Findings bore this out, in that invalid male patients were more likely than women to be sent to Tranquillity's sick ward, which was notably run by female nursing staff. This suggests that the intimacies and obligations of familial ties were heavily reinforced by gender stereotypic considerations, dictating that care work is particularly appropriate to women, and in this context to women patients.

In addition to ward-based chores, occupational therapy was offered to long-stay patients at Tranquillity, although this felicitous wording suggests that patients could freely choose to participate without coercion, which I would certainly not suggest was the case. Long-stay patients were in fact targeted for occupational therapy, due to the perception that this could be of little value to recently admitted acute cases, who were expected to merely sit out the duration of their stay on the wards. Occupational work at Tranquillity, therefore, was traditionally seen as an important way of keeping otherwise idle hands employed, while contributing to the hospital revenue and highly reminiscent of the kinds of employment that would have been encouraged among asylum patients in the nineteenth century colonial asylums in Malaya and India. This being the case, chronic patients would normally be allocated whatever work was available, as this medical assistant pointed out,

> *(There is) insufficient analysis of social needs - no matching of interests to the work ... Chronic patients have no say in what they do ... they obey the staff ... What choice do they have?*

Anthropologists often claim that although different in kind, the work performed by men and women in Southeast Asia is usually of a complementary nature, and is relatively equal in importance between the sexes (Appell, 1991; Monnig Atkinson, 1990; Rousseau, 1991). At Hospital Tranquillity occupational therapy was also divided into work considered suitable for men and women respectively, but here the types of work performed by men and women were clearly distinguishable in terms of status and reward. This situation was reminiscent of traditional asylum care where activities were highly gender specific and frequently revolved around those that required physical exertion (Rutherford, 2008). In the UK husbandry on the land and making coconut fibre mats, for example, tended to usefully expend energy that might otherwise be more harmfully (or less productively) released, and was furthermore considered to be morally and emotionally beneficial. In a modern Malaysian context male patients, for example, were able to participate in carpentry, basket weaving[1] and farming activities, which took place on a small scale in the hospital grounds. Women were occupied solely with craft work, which consisted basically of repetitive work using fabric, and given handicraft tasks to do dependent on their skills and levels of concentration. Once again, in common with the factory setting, women were easily allocated the least-skilled and most unstimulating tasks possible, that of the deft but prolonged extraction of threads from scraps of cloth (Ong, 1990). This 'thread-sorting' activity was seen to be particularly suitable for women psychiatric patients and was incredibly tedious work that usually took place at long trestle tables on the ward. The end result was that the piles of individual threads were used as stuffing material for a small range of household goods, manufactured by staff and other patients in the occupational therapy department. This situation is highly reminiscent of descriptions of patient labour in Victorian asylums, such as those that involved picking out lumps in horsehair destined to be used as stuffing for bed mattresses (Rutherford, 2008).

By contrast, with the predominant activity for women, male patients were given the opportunity to apply their skills in carpentry, producing sturdy and creditable pieces for sale. The basketry department produced an array of smaller items and larger pieces of rattan furniture; most of these items were usually sold to kindergartens in town, which held a contract with the hospital. Finally, male chronic patients were also involved in small-scale gardening activities, with the chronic wards producing leafy vegetables, most of which was sold to staff. *Bunga Raya* ward had taken advantage of the expertise of many of its rural-born patients and had developed an enviable specialist activity, providing a good deal of independence for those involved in the activity. This was livestock farming, predominantly a business in breeding quails, chickens and goats, and which appeared to provide a small but steady income. Like that from all other such activities this was ploughed back into the hospital revenues under the 'Patients' Fund' from which patient salaries were deducted. Earnings on the forensic ward were some of the highest obtainable in this system, and the work was comparatively stimulating and autonomous.

In reference to colonial Africa and the British Raj both Jackson (2005) and Ernst (2010) note that physical occupations, like farming, were undertaken by indigenous patients, rather than their white counterparts, where in the latter case at least, physical exertion was considered too taxing for the colonial patients. However, Jackson (2005) implies that these tasks were imposed a deliberate form of hard labour as a demeaning demarcation of the Africans' racial inferiority. In contrast to this farming was clearly a high status occupation for male patients at Tranquillity. It also conformed to a traditional model that retains much political and ideological currency in Malaysia in reinforcing the dual values of an individualistic and collective work ethic in patients, as an unqualified benefit for both patients and the institution (Deva, 2004).

Skilled work undertaken by the men therefore could potentially command a relatively good income by the standards of the hospital, as Abang on Male Ward 1 pointed out,

Abang:	Yes, I am hardworking. Last time (before an admission) I was farming over there, digging holes, clearing grass, building houses and moving a gas stove.
Researcher:	What about in here?
Abang:	At the time of Dr Abdul (previous director of the hospital) he didn't ask me to go to the carpentry. I just stay here all the time but when Dr Siong took over, he asked me to go there. Maybe it's good because I can earn some money, even if not much.
Researcher:	And you learn new skills?
Abang:	No, I just polish the wood.
Researcher:	Do you make furniture?
Abang:	Yes, it is hard work. I don't make furniture, I polish the wood and sometimes I take the tools that we need from the store. I get a salary from going to carpentry. At first they said they will give us RM [ringgit Malaysia] 8.00 a month but we get around RM 20 each month. I was surprised!

Occupational work undertaken by men and women differed not only in the levels of skill required, with women relegated to largely unskilled and highly monotonous activities, but this was also reflected in the token earnings that patients achieved based on sales. Handicrafts paid the least under the present regime, resulting in women patients being subjected to a replication of the economic inequalities inherent in conventional patriarchal, capitalistic societies as well as being rife with gender stereotyping (Wetzel, 2000; Witz, 1992).

> Occupational-therapy programmes gave many patients a sense of dignity, with a renewed interest in life, but they also reflected a rigid and Victorian stereotype of gender perhaps more than any aspect of hospital life (Gittins, 1998: 107).

Ah Ming, for example, was a multiply admitted woman who had unusually been given a factory-type punch card by Dr Jerry, one of the few psychiatrists at the hospital, ensuring that a certain number of hours were devoted to the work. Her role at home was that of an impoverished, aging spinster sister reliant on the unwilling charity of the family. As the 'poor relative' she acted as an unpaid if somewhat unreliable domestic servant, but more than this her diagnosis marked her out for exclusion as a pariah. An angry woman, her resentment occasionally resulted in violent quarrels with family members in which Ah Ming tended to come off the worst, followed by a prompt readmission to hospital. At Tranquillity, the rigorous training Ah Ming was subjected to through the punch-card system seemed designed to discipline her into uncomplaining, ill-paid, unfulfilling and mind-numbingly tedious work compatible with her stigmatised station in life as a woman with a psychiatric history. When this was accomplished to the satisfaction of staff, she would be considered fit for discharge back to the dubious care of her family.

Rehabilitative work for women at Tranquillity was undoubtedly remarkably lacking in stimulation, as well as being financially and personally unrewarding. This raises some serious questions about the nature of such 'therapeutic' activities and what kinds of messages were being reinforced to patients through forms of exploitation premised upon sexist and capitalistic practices. On the wards, however, through the normative employment of familial connections between patients, women's labour became an equally valuable commodity to be utilised. Yet in this respect exploitation was to some degree allayed, as by the nature of things this tended to compensate some patients through offering the personal benefits of bonding with one another.

The enclosed world of the total institution imposes its own logic upon routines, rationale and interpersonal morphologies. However, for those sequestered at Hospital Tranquillity, the regulated social existence of life in the asylum reflects the hierarchies of influence that merely replicate in a distorted form the 'civic' world beyond the walls. The bizarre mirroring of the external world at the Hospital decreases incrementally as an observer acquaints themself with the diverse enactments of autonomy and control by patients and staff moving in their singular and occasionally colliding orbits.

Note

1   Among the Selako people of Sarawak, however, basket weaving is considered a feminine activity (Schneider and Schneider, 1991: 349).

6
Healing, medication and resistance

Historically advances in medical treatment in the area of psychiatry have been read in terms of social advances for the greater benefit of the public (Shorter, 1997). Yet treatment and medication are not neutral or invariably positive activities and for many psychiatric dissenters they are viewed as issues of hegemonic power and control, as well as of individual resistance (O'Hagan, 1996; Szasz, 1974). Fennell, for example, draws attention to the means by which non-voluntary psychiatric treatment has been sanitised, and brought into a general public acceptance through appeals to the common good.

> The common feature of these medical breakthroughs was that they were often performed for the greater good and greater glory of medicine, on patients who were incapable of consenting or who adamantly refused them, and who were certainly never told of the likely effects (Fennell, 1996: 139).

The implication is that the beneficial effects of medical care must occasionally therefore be imposed for the good of the patient through control. Busfield, however, points out that if the discourse of 'control' is counterbalanced by that of 'care' then this constitutes a false dichotomy.

> Care and control in mental health services .... are not, however, mutually exclusive alternatives ... for control is integral to caring. (Busfield, 1996a: 233).

Resistance to treatment, however, is often interpreted in terms of pathology in psychiatric patients, which in turn defines them more clearly as being in need of *management* for *appropriate* care to be administered (Estroff, 1981). At Hospital Tranquillity staff largely regarded treatment as devoid of political or ideological nuances. Rather, it was seen in a matter-of-fact light, to the extent that medication administration, as well as medical assessments and resulting discussions on the subject, took place publicly on the open ward, providing the occasional distracting interlude to an otherwise mundane hour. If confidentiality was not regarded as an issue for consideration on the wards, neither was user participation encouraged in the interrogation of patients by professionals, as this observed account demonstrates.

Field notes. Female Ward 1.

The doctor on duty is examining cases, patients are called over to him but he barely raises his head to look at them. The nurses play the part of both informant and attendant. Now and again questions are asked of the patient in a mixture of English and Bahasa Malayu. But this isn't an interactive session as such: the nurses gather round the doctor to provide information that may be confirmed by the patient or alternatively display the patient's level of dysfunction, as in the case of the 'defaulter'.

This is a very apathetic Chinese woman, her body slumped, head bowed, face almost expressionless. Getting her to say anything is an effort. She is introduced to the doctor: 'This one is a defaulter'. A moral judgement is passed immediately. A brief discussion between doctor and nurses ensues with additional information provided: 'the husband is very supportive'. A brief question is posed to the patient and not answering immediately, she is prodded by a nurse into replying. One nurse demonstrates the patient's confusion by asking, 'how many children have you got, eh? How many? Four, yes? *Empat!* (four)'. She nods feebly. The interrogation continues, 'how old are they your children?' Apparently the patient gets the answer wrong and is told so. Of her own volition the patient attempts to add some more information but this is not required apparently. A nurse smacks her arm impatiently and she lapses once again into silence. Another comments, '..the husband is very ambitious – studying MBA (Masters of Business Administration) in his own time!' The doctor and nurse gaze at the patient with some amazement, as if wondering how such a wreck could attract and keep the devotion of clearly a high flier.

Medication defaulting was therefore considered to be the main reason for 'revolving door' admissions, and consequently a continuous area of conflict between exasperated staff and recalcitrant patients, who once discharged to their own community were free to follow their own inclination. Outpatient groups like these were nominally catered for by the community psychiatric nursing programme (CPN). The implementation of the CPNs at the hospital has been justified primarily in terms of being an effective weapon in the prevention of medication defaulting amongst outpatients, and only secondly as providing a community service aimed at meeting the needs of those unable to access outpatient facilities regularly (Lau and Hardin, 1996). Consequently, how compliant a patient was seen to be became a measure by which to judge an individual's personal worth, as well as prognosis. Rarely, however, was this used as a means of evaluating the method of treatment itself, a move which Arthur Kleinman interprets as implying the 'moral hegemony' of medical science over that of personal meaning and autonomy (Fadiman 1997: 261).

Within the ward setting little tolerance was shown towards patients who refused to accept their medication willingly. This uncompromising professional attitude towards refusal was unclear to me at the beginning of fieldwork; and so naively, being well informed of Western service-user critiques of medication, I was somewhat surprised to find that this was not a burning issue of contention that patients were willing to raise with me in discussion. Instead, patients at Tranquillity appeared to view medication as a normal and mundane part of their daily routines. In support of this apparent disinterest, I noted that, at least in my presence, very few patients of either sex offered anything approaching resistance at medication time. On the locked ward in Male Ward 1, for instance, given the command people presented themselves at the bars to seemingly compliantly ingest pills or offer arms ready for jabs, without even inconveniencing the staff into unlocking the grill gate. Eventually, however, I began to uncover indications that some patients were in fact quite suspicious of the perceived deleterious effects of medication upon their metabolism, as Geranting on Female Ward 1 commented.

It's weird that everyone here is sleepy and weak after taking medication. It may be good but it makes people so weak, and always sleeping.

On the private wards by contrast, ex-serviceman Abdul Mohammed, rather relished the spaced-out feeling created by medication, which he described as a pleasant *berkhayal* (daydreaming). Boon Chieng, the *prominent* on Male Ward 1, was flatly opposed (although outwardly 'compliant') to taking his medication, due mostly to these debilitating side effects, and was understandably highly suspicious of the way his medication was altered now and again without any explanation. Ironically, although medication was being used to tackle his paranoid schizophrenia, this situation inadvertently served to feed his dreadful fantasies further.

These views collectively are reflected in turn by those of service users in the UK, where Rogers *et al.* (1993: 122), and separately Barham and Hayward (1996), note concerns regarding the loss of energy and unpleasant side effects brought about by the use of tranquillisers and anti-psychotic drugs. Jonathan Gabe (1996: 188), however, might appreciate Abdul Mohammed's point of view, in commenting on research that indicates the value users placed on the soothing 'peace of mind' created through the use of medication. Julie Leibrich in turn draws on her own experience as a service user when she describes her ambivalence towards medication,

> Once or twice they have saved my life, but they also numb me and make it harder for me to connect with my spirit. So in the long run, they make it harder to heal (Leibrich, 2002: 149).

In the best spirit of ethnographic exploration, Sue Estroff bravely self-administers Prolixin hydrochloride, in order to experience the effect personally. Having encountered a variety of unpleasantly disorientating side-effects she concludes her experiment with relief, and little surprise at the negative responses towards medication amongst her user participants (Estroff, 1981).

However, at Tranquillity a level of acceptance of medication on the wards was demonstrated to the extent that patients for the most part accepted pills and injections as a routine that they had to adjust to, even if this was not much liked, as obliquely indicated in this comment by a long-stay patient.

> *Getting up? There's no particular time, nothing is fixed except taking ubat (medicine) and chores maybe. People don't always get up at the same time because they may be knocked out by ubat.*

Patients who had been 'knocked out' by medication were accordingly a normal sight on the ward, to which little attention was generally paid, as indicated in the following observation taken from field notes.

Field notes. Male Ward 1.

Today, unusually for this ward, I found a patient tied to his bed - this is a large Chinese man snoring soundly and secured firmly, absolutely oblivious to the noise on the ward. Apparently a new admission and not yet seen by the ward doctor, according to the MA on duty. He (the patient) has spent the first night screaming and shouting, necessitating tranquillisers and now restraints, to stop him falling off the bed.

Coercion was another recognised fact of life on the wards and the pragmatic acceptance of medication by patients tended to conceal the repercussions that awaited a show of real resistance. On one occasion, I witnessed the results of patient resistance in which a woman in the locked section had been refusing to take her medication for hours and so it was decided that it would have to be given by force. Four nurses entered into the locked section and pinned her face down on the bed, whilst another injected her in the buttock despite her screams, and then quickly withdrew. Under these circumstances then patients were more likely to openly accept medication rather than suffer the oppressive consequences of refusal. As Desjarlais (1996) notes of service users in his Boston study there is a significant and crucial difference in the position between not wanting to take medication in general and refusing one's prescribed drugs in view of the consequences of refusal. This therefore tends to lead to a high degree of ambivalence towards the very act of being compliant (Desjarlais, 1996).

Over time, I found that the responses given by participants became more complex and insightful as in my interviews with Petrus, a teenage first-admission male patient enduring his first spell in the locked section of Male Ward 1. Initially when we discussed the subject of medication in a semi-formal interview his comments seemed blasé and superficial in keeping with his laconic, worldly air and he professed to have no particular antipathy towards the unknown injections and pills regularly administered.

Some weeks following his discharge, I doggedly tracked Petrus down for another conversation at the golf course café where he was doing casual work. He seemed a very different person on this encounter. Thoroughly amused to see me he was positively elated by his new-found freedom, radiant and intoxicated with freedom, he had a very different account to give this time.

Researcher:	Did the hospital give you medicines to take when you were discharged?
Petrus:	Yes, three packets, and I was to come back for more when I was finished. But I haven't finished them yet.
Researcher:	Were you meant to take them every day?
Petrus:	Yes, but I only take them when I've got a headache.
Researcher:	Do you know what they are for? Did they (staff) explain what they for?
Petrus:	They only said that if I take them I'll be well. But I am well now so I only take them when I feel ill.
Researcher:	Although you are meant to take them every day, aren't you?
Petrus:	Yes

Researcher:	So …?
Petrus:	I don't like taking *ubat*.
Researcher:	Why is that?
Petrus:	Why don't I like taking them? (Pause) Maybe because I don't want to be part of that system. If you take *ubat* then everyone thinks you must be ill – I am not ill. (Pause) It's good to be out of that place, I don't like being told what to do.

As Estroff points out, this kind of argument contains its own logic: only sick people take medication, therefore to constantly take medication is to constantly advertise sickness to oneself and others, and therefore suffer the deprivation of a hope of recovery (Estroff, 1981: 112). Petrus felt well at that time, effectively he felt 'cured' of some distressing symptoms, and therefore there was no need to take medication, despite staff providing the usual information, namely that his condition was only 'treatable' not 'curable'. Furthermore, Petrus did not really know what the medications did biochemically and did not much care, but made it clear that he was unwilling to accept a life of being constantly defined as sick, with the subsequent control by health authorities that such status implied. Needless to say, Petrus's attitude would be censured by the hospital staff as 'non-compliant' and as an indication of his lack of insight, which in itself is seen as symptomatic of schizophrenia.

Unpleasant side effects caused by tranquillisers, anti-depressants and anti-psychotic drugs apart, the stigma and the sense of hopelessness caused by continuous use of medication appeared to be good reasons for medication defaulting once the opportunity presented. At Tranquillity, patient anxieties about the side effects of drugs were not frequently acknowledged as a serious concern by ward staff, but was at least duly noted by the hospital director. He was candid in describing the more serious side effects caused by anti-psychotic drugs, such as tardive dyskinesia, as well as the lesser effects of drowsiness, constipation and a dry mouth, as a definite disincentive. Since in his opinion so many patients must take these medications for life, the side effects of medication were practically never discussed with patients beforehand for fear of alarming them and their families, an omission that, as he said, is practised 'in other countries'. Presumably, the assumption by staff was that the evidence of side effects manifested by other patients around them would be passed off as an individual peculiarity, rather than the sad consequence of side effects. This presumption would seem to be an optimistic one in that, judging from patients' comments, side effects were not merely a known but feared outcome of compliance.

Healing and Spirituality

Despite a growing professional and academic interest in forms of spirituality, religious fervour is often perceived to be uncontainable, where it is feared that the boundaries of reason are easily transgressed and zeal degenerates into mere expressions of madness. In her exploration of the peak of religious madness in nineteenth century Germany, Goldberg (1999) comments on the different attitudes early French and German alienists held towards the issue of the Church, religion and insanity. For Pinel and his ilk the association of clericism with royalism, versus a rationalist paradigm would dictate the need to reject the role of the Church in the emerging science of psychiatry (Goldberg, 1999). By contrast, German counterparts were more closely allied to the Church, and thereby viewed religion 'as a bulwark against mental and social disorder' (Goldberg, 1999: 48).

In Malaysia adherence to a religion continues to define a social norm; and the anti-clericism that has been a feature of many European countries from the eighteenth century holds little sway in this region. Yet here too a power struggle has been enacted to divest the various arms of organised religion in this country of the care and cure of the insane. The division between the domains and authority of psychiatry and that of religion is clearly marked in professional circles, but not so easily demarcated among the patient population or the communities from which they have emerged, as the following accounts from psychiatric patients will serve to illustrate.

A useful starting point to consider the issue of mental distress and religious/spiritual personal interpretations from the service user point of view is provided by Leibrich (2002), who reflects upon her personal perspective of recovery. This lies in the acceptance of the illness and the use of this experience as a means of discovering a spiritual dimension that must come to the fore to enable real healing to take place. Insight and self-knowledge emerge from this struggle and develop into a sense of wholeness that opposes a threatened fracture of self (Leibrich, 2002).

> It is increasingly understood that psychotherapists' views of humanity directly and indirectly affect how they view disorders and struggles, and consequently how he or she understands growth and healing (Howard *et al.*, 2000: 309).

Likewise, several patients at Tranquillity seemed to be engaged in just this endeavour of seeking spiritual unity in the effort to regain equilibrium. Tuyah for example, as a self-appointed *dukun*, and Jacob, as a proclaimed Christian, were resigned to taking medication, whilst actually dedicating themselves in private to their own personal healing rituals (Lewis, 1996). Foo, a quiet, devout Buddhist youth spent much time reading as well as practising meditation, energy devoted to spiritual development being seen as essential in the slow progress towards recovery. Edward, another fervent Christian, described his compulsory admission to hospital as a personal test of worth, as well as time in retreat, much as a monk might view a time of solitude as testing and sacred.

> *After being here I feel the Holy Spirit is trying to find out whether I am fit for the task. ..Now I feel I have received the message. It is all within me. Only at this moment I feel weak (physically) but my thinking is always strong....At this moment God has not shown me the way to start my work. He has only asked me to wait for the time to arrive...I have a feeling of both fear and happiness, but most of all immense joy.*

The working compromise these patients offered was to pay a nominal lip service to the reputed benefits of biomedicine for the sake of peace, whilst in fact having a far greater faith in their own therapeutic regimes. These personal regimes towards health were plans that the ward staff appeared to either generally unaware of, or did not accept as credible strategies (Oldnall, 1996; McSherry, 1998; Younger, 1995).

While many of the more bizarre religious experiences voiced by patients could easily be dismissed by staff as psychotic outpourings, others appeared to emanate from genuine commitment.

> These people are guided by traditional wisdom that sees illness as a disorder of the whole person who is not divided into body and mind and is in close relation to the cosmos and the deities (Fernando, 2010: 80)

Faith, as Roger Fallot (2001) points out, engenders feelings of self-respect and endurance, reducing stress and conferring integrity and meaning onto the otherwise demeaning experience of being a psychiatric patient. If, however, fragmentation is the feared result of mental disorder, and a sense of wholeness the therapeutic goal, it indicates that the professionals involved in their care needed to take into account the patient's sense of spiritual self, instead of focusing on the 'mechanics' of the job (Greasley *et al.*, 2001: 629).

Here Acharyya's point (1996), followed by Fernando (2010), is well taken, in arguing that psychiatry dislocates Western-trained psychiatrists from their own cultural milieu, while Fallot (2001) goes on to suggest that therefore an important step could be taken through collaboration with traditional healers and spiritual advisors. In cultures like Malaysia, where the use of traditional healing methods is as commonplace as that of biomedicine, this would seem a pragmatic and culturally apposite way to proceed. Whether there is a class element attached to belief systems that are culturally grounded, in addition to issues of ethnicity in Malaysia, requires further research, but it is apparent that class influences interpretation and decision-making in contemporary India, although rich in respected healing traditions (Wagner *et al.*, 1999). Nevertheless, in reference to Malaysia, this is not to suggest that traditional healing methods stand in opposed unity to biomedicine.

A new strand of tension also exists in terms of traditional beliefs and the established religions of Islam and Christianity in Malaysia. Although the *bomoh* is a central healing figure in pre-Islamic culture this is a marginalized role in Islam. Nonetheless, a strong belief in the existence of the supernatural is far from being eroded: as recently as 1986 an Islamic court on Peninsular Malaysia fined a woman for adultery with an incubus (Gullick, 1987; Lewis, 1995). Furthermore, diverse Christian sects and healing rituals flourished in this region following the evangelical enterprises of competing missionaries. The results are that eclectic visions of cure and Christianity pepper the narratives of individuals.

Finally, which religion or sect was the more effective in terms of curative powers, was a lively if perplexing topic amongst patient participants of all cultural backgrounds. This flexible lack of orthodox adherence to a particular belief system conforms with Fernando's (2010: 147) description of the benefits to psychiatric service users in South India of being able to 'shop around' among a range of therapies, including those offered at a Muslim mosque, Hindu temple and Christian church.

Despite these diverse beliefs, and the numbers of patients who continued to seek traditional healing in plurality with psychiatry, the hospital had no intention of initiating any form of open collaboration with healers. By contrast, Jackson (2005) describes how postcolonial Zimbabwe has warmly encouraged the participation of traditional healers in the care of the mentally ill, as a powerful form of indigenisation and gesture of decolonisation, Moreover, in the West, cult adoption of diverse traditional healing forms, from Native American traditions to Tibetan Buddhist disciplines, to name but two, testify to the need by sufferers, disenchanted with biomedical approaches, to seek alternative, spiritually grounded forms of relief (Fernando, 2010).

The issue of whether the medical model and traditional healing practices represent competing or overlapping paradigms is a moot point where the aggressive dominance of biomedicine could be quite clearly seen at Tranquillity. Although staff might, for instance, seek traditional healing practices for their own needs, being seen to encourage or at least tolerate this kind of health-seeking behaviour by patients was tantamount to bringing the psychiatric profession into disrepute. That being overtly the case, covertly staff might empathise with the wish to obtain help from traditional healers, according to the account given to me by Mr Song, a most well-respected *dang ke* (Chinese traditional healer) practising locally, who claimed that amongst his many clients some were patients at Tranquillity.

Clad in red and white, with a sash tied round his head like a kamikaze pilot, Mr Song conducted his practice in the main room of his suburban house, which was dramatically decorated with the paraphernalia of ceremony: symbols, statues and an overpowering smell of incense. Here he treated a variety of complaints across generations brought to him by conventionally diagnosed patients and others, even including some medical staff. With psychiatric patients the dilemma was to distinguish between genuine mental illness, spirit possession, or some other kind of illness understood within the cultural schema. These kinds of cases were occasionally referred through advice, rather than prescription, from concerned medical personnel when noting that little progress has been made towards eliminating 'hysterical' (psychotic) attacks in otherwise fairly rational individuals. Later, uniformed in his sober city day dress and spectacles Mr Song, calm and candid, was willing, without any show of defensiveness, to discuss in a learned manner his methods and conclusions.

In cases like these doctors need to understand that the illness cannot be cured or treated by medication. It needs other help to send the spirits away – and maybe also through counselling. When doctors come across these kinds of patients they realise that a spiritual world does exist. The only problem is, it cannot be proved. It is only if you see for yourself then you would believe it'

Mr. Song, like many other traditional healers in this region, worked across cultural boundaries, both ethnic and ideological. *Puan* (Madam) Junita, for example, was an Iban *manang*, a healer and spirit medium of some fame who normally plied her trade from her home in a traditional longhouse in the rural outback. Introduced to her by a friendly longhouse retinue, I found her a taciturn individual who was willing to grant me only a brief audience as we sat on the rush mats that carpeted the floor of her *bilik* (longhouse cabin). In the deep gloom of this barn-like, spartanly furnished space her slight silhouette was more easily seen than her features. This, and her air of being only tenuously tied to this time and place, preserved her mystery. Doling out her words thriftily she claimed to have worked with many different people in her time, including those with formally diagnosed mental illnesses, although with varying levels of success. In the best tradition she inherited her paranormal skills from a grandparent, becoming acquainted with her vocation only by undergoing the physical and mental crisis that leads to insight and rebirth as a medium. This crisis, as hospitalised Tuyah knew, is not dissimilar on the face of it to a mental breakdown; however, the outcome could not be further removed from the stigmatised role of incurable, social outcast, as experienced by most psychiatric patients in developed nations (Silverman, 1967).

Surrounded by the tools of daily living, as well as those of her trade, *Puan* Junita warmed briefly to the subject and her audience, explaining that most of her patients had visited and been disappointed by conventional doctors before coming to see her. For her part, patients could be successfully helped provided that theirs was, for example, a case of broken *pantang* (taboo) and consequent possession by a *hantu* (ghost or spirit). If the condition was inherited, her success rate was less impressive. However, each patient was assessed individually, and with due professionalism she refused to generalise further on her ability to help others without first seeing them in person.

In his study on spirit possession and shamans I.M. Lewis (1995) argues that anthropologists have traditionally been antagonistic towards psychiatry, preferring to locate normative differences in conduct within cultural interpretation. In this vein Sindzingre discusses illness and explanation among the Senufo of the Ivory Coast, stating that the medical model views illness as devoid of 'intentionality', where illness in general has no special meaning or particular significance (1995: 74). In relation to psychiatry and psychology, this probably overstates the case, as the patient's frames of reference are usually of interest to mental health professionals, if only to determine levels of mental abnormality. Loustaunau and Sobo (1997: 108) make the point that biomedicine itself in merely a cultural construct, although one that is so dominant as to form a conventional yardstick by which to measure other healing approaches.

Culture, however, is a central locus of the individual, and just as Tuyah regards her symptoms as tokens of her shamanistic destiny, other patients at Tranquillity interpret their states of mind or time spent in the hospital as symbolic of something other and far greater than a desiccated medical label denoting mental illness. Waxler (1997) suggests that the prognosis of illness in the individual cultural context dramatically influences the course and outcome of illness. In developing countries 'sanctions or activities' carried out by traditional healers, for instance, become an opportunity for group participation and assimilation of the afflicted individual. It is interesting to note that in reference to the Iban *Dayaks* of Sarawak, Schmidt (1964) describes this precise process, which serves as a form of re-assertion of community cohesiveness.

The other side of the coin indicates, as Warner points out, that the protective factors of social integration in themselves militate against the powerful effects of stigma (1996). When abnormal behaviours are viewed not so much in terms of individual deviance but are reframed within a cultural interpretation, where the sufferer is the innocent victim of supernatural aetiologies or circumstance, blame and stigma are more likely to be suspended (Fidler, 1993).

> In reference to culpability and stigma the explanation of supramundane causality tended to exculpate sufferers, who were now no longer seen as *orang gila* (madmen) but as innocent victims of *orang buat* (sorceror/witch). From this perspective the explanation served to relieve the sufferer and his/her family from social censure and normative measures could now be undertaken to exorcise the malign spirit through ceremony and ritual (Ashencaen Crabtree and Chong, 1999a).

Under these circumstances, it is therefore not surprising to find that the prognosis of individuals is much improved in many Third World countries, where a low level of stigma is attached to mental disorders, in possible combination with traditional healing remedies (Sartorius *et al.*, 1977). Yet in the Malaysian context stigma towards mental illness undoubtedly exists, despite flourishing cultures of traditional healing; and especially where aggressive or sexually deviant behaviour might accompany bizarre but innocuous behaviour (Warner, 1996; Ashencaen Crabtree, 1999a).

Many patients, regardless of sex, evidently did not feel that they were in a position to protest against treatment following admission, and it is arguable how far patients could be seen to have given their genuine consent to treatment in the first place. Whether staff felt that treatment given by force damaged their day-to-day relationships with patients is unclear, although evidence from a survey of British service users conducted by People First indicates that patients perceived this as causing a serious breach of trust (Rogers and Pilgrim, 1992; Rogers *et al.*, 1993). In terms of ward control at Tranquillity, however, the use of medication, and ECT in particular, played a vital role in maintaining order whilst being upheld as benign and therapeutic.

ECT as an instrument of control

On Female Ward 1, relationships with some informants were marked by an increase in the depth and types of confidences shared, which gave me further insight into medication and treatment that patients found particularly disturbing. Of more consequence to these women than the general administration and side effects of the usual kinds of *ubat*, notably tranquillisers and anti-psychotic drugs, was the routine administration of electro-convulsive therapy (ECT), as suggested in this extract from field notes.

Field notes. Female Ward 1.

On the ward, nothing much happening, except that I see a woman in the locked section with a large gauze plaster on her chin being escorted out of the ward by some nurses. Behind them a nurse wheels a wheelchair - it's obvious she is on her way to ECT. I ask the patients and they confirm this – it's amazing that so many of them have had ECT repeatedly ….

Later, on the way out I see a nurse wheeling the woman I saw earlier back to the ward. The nurse is moving briskly and in the chair the woman doesn't look much the worse for wear except for a fixed and wide-eyed stare. We pass each other without any change in her frozen regard.

Jane Ussher (1991) contends that women in modern Britain have been subject to ECT in increasingly high numbers and are, in fact, more likely to be subjected to this form of treatment than men. Hospital records at Tranquillity are unable to quantify the use of ECT in the patient population, or to corroborate a ratio in relation to gender variables, yet ECT does seem to be in common practice at the hospital based on the accounts given by patients and staff (Rack, 1982). Thus, given the helpful cue from women patients I was then able to take this issue back into the male wards for further discussion with patients, and seemingly stumbled on a topic that generated a good deal of anxiety, and indeed fear, amongst patients.

ECT has of course received a notorious press, although there are many service users in Britain who have equally found it to be highly beneficial (Kesey, 1962; Perkins, 1996; Rogers *et al.*, 1993; Taylor, 1996). ECT at Hospital Tranquillity was used for a diverse range of patients, rather than being dedicated to the treatment of 'serious, intractable depression' to describe its conventional use by Rogers *et al.* (1993: 123; World Health Organization, 1997). In interview, Dr Tiong Mee Siew was very candid about the use of ECT in the hospital, saying that it used to be applied 'indiscriminately' in the past. This observation echoes past accounts of the use of ECT in French colonial psychiatric hospitals in North Africa, where all manner of the latest curative treatments were available for use on Maghrebian patients, including lumbar punctures, 'cocktails of mercury, arsenic and cyanide', insulin shocks and ECT (Keller, 2007: 28). Keller goes on to controversially add that the uses and abuses of ECT in the Maghreb may have paved the way for electrical shock as a tool of torture during the later Algerian war.

At Tranquillity during these more enlightened times ECT was used more specifically; however it was not retained just for its conventional usage but operated on a wider client group. Due to staff shortages and the lack of individual secure units, ECT at Tranquillity was imposed on those patients deemed to be exhibiting problematic behaviour on the ward, such as general disruption and aggression and therefore:

> *This settles their behaviour very quickly and makes them more manageable. So ECT in this way overcomes our nursing problems.*

For the director this use of ECT was far from ideal, yet the overcrowding on the ward coupled with insufficient numbers of supervisory staff, dictated that a somewhat draconian level of control would be in operation at times. Consequently, ECT has been maintained as a very effective means of managing patients' behaviour and is duly reminiscent of similar accounts of its use in colonial Fiji during the 1940s, where ECT was used to 'settle ... mind and body', coupled with the increasing introduction of psychotropic drugs (Leckie, 2007: 115). This method of behavioural control, however, needs to be balanced by evidence of the use of psychosurgery, such as leucotomies and lobotomies, where in relation to Southern Rhodesia in 1946 twenty such operations had been performed on mostly African female patients with behavioural problems' with results that a report of the time described as having 'gratifying' results (McCulloch, 1995:19). This, however, was a highly limited experiment compared to the many thousands who underwent lobotomy in the United States by 1951 (Sacks, 1995). Jackson (2005), however, considers the method of administration of ECT in South Rhodesia, which, as was commonly the case in the 1940s, was not preceded by anaesthesia for patients in general. Nevertheless, it is claimed that this practice continued into the late 1950s on African patients solely at the Ingutsheni Mental Hospital (Jackson, 2005).

In relation to the use of ECT at Tranquillity, how liberal a contemporary regime these modernised practices represents, in comparison with the procedures of twenty and thirty years ago, can be gauged by the following extracts from field notes.

Field notes. Male Ward 1.

T.P. a long-serving, authoritative MA is happy to discuss changes he has seen in the hospital during his long career here. He describes various horrors, such as the condition in the locked wards, and ECT as it was conducted in the past where the patients were fully conscious and terrified.

They (patients) had to be dragged to the machines and the staff would go around the ward shocking them, sometimes about 20 people all around the room. It was terrible. It was torture – torturing the patients ... But then I think it was the Americans stopped that - ECT without anaesthesia - some rules were made... It was also terrible for the staff as well of course.

Frankie from Bunga Raya ward has spent most of his life in psychiatric care and recalled the past clearly. Frankie was a useful source of personal information on ECT treatment and was able to provide a personal account that fit the descriptions provided by the medical assistant, albeit from a very different position:

I had it (ECT) many times, many times. Terrible experience – ECT. Terrible experience! Like fire in my head – electric current. [Frankie holds both sides of his forehead with his fingers] *So fast. Terrible.*

Frankie indicates that he was awake at the time but that the sessions rendered him unconscious. He goes on to explain why he received ECT.

To calm me down. I was always standing up ... But thank the Lord all well, so calm now ... it's not practical in a hospital to stand up like that. Yes, I was calmer after .... I was unconscious for hours. During those times yes, I was very ... nervous.'

It remains unclear exactly how long ECT was practised in this kind of fashion, and it is therefore just as difficult to ascertain when more humane procedures were brought in at Hospital Tranquillity, and understandably ward staff are reticent about being seen to criticise previous management.

Although it is quite clear that things have improved considerably at the hospital, some patients interviewed were far from happy about being subjected to the procedure. Burly, good natured Dimbaud from Male Ward 1 received ECT once, and was so appalled by the subsequent memory losses which he experienced sporadically 'for five months!' that when ECT was suggested to him once again upon a further admission he broke out of the hospital somehow and made his escape.

Patrick, a nervous young Chinese man on Male Ward 1 was full of trepidation, as on the following day he was scheduled to receive his first course of ECT at his mother's instigation, which he quite clearly resented deeply. As a Catholic, he had asked his local priest for guidance, but since his priest concurred with his mother, Patrick was willing to reluctantly submit to the feared treatment. Patrick evidently attempted to view this in a spirit of Christian humility arising maybe from a mixture of anger, hopelessness, helplessness and maybe a desire to please.

Some people sacrifice their bodies, but others also choose to sacrifice their minds.

On Female Ward 1 Aini, my droll, eloquent Malay informant gave a lyrical yet graphic account of her experience of ECT treatment.

When not well - when mind is chronic – your speaking not a structure – imagine things – hearing voices. ECT – with a current all over your head and a wire in your hand – a needle in your hand …. Vibrations of sound make us giddy - it radiates the mind in circulation… First an injection is given, half asleep, half aware – feeling of something afloat – drifting slowly and slowly – fast asleep. Like a thunder moving with a storm. Like a sea breeze with the wave …. Very painful and giddy [holding temples] vomiting - under our chest got pain… When I got my third ECT this year, when I was 36 (years old) - I was awake 25 minutes …

[I am uncertain what Aini means when she says she was 'awake' as she also says she was under anaesthetic, i.e. 'asleep'].

Researcher:	Can you remember afterwards?
Aini:	Not yet actually …We remember things, slowly remember.
Researcher:	Do you think ECT is a good sort of medication?
Aini:	Not very good, ECT. Sometimes destroys our organic systems.
Soo Mei:	If I am unhappy, it makes you feel more happy, but cannot help you.

Aini:	Sometimes you remember - sometimes you forget - like waves.
Maria:	Bad memory. ECT no good, bad memory. 6 times! (Received ECT). Pills better.
Tuyah:	Whole body shaking – electricalised.

Whether staff were aware of how their patients felt about the treatments available at the hospital, the position of staff on the benefits of medication was, as would be expected, largely unanimous. While force was seen as an inconvenient and unpleasant duty, it was nonetheless regarded as necessary to retain order. Although medical assistant Tua regarded ECT as being a 'cruel' sort of treatment yet he continued to administer it, and said in its defence that there was no doubt that some people appeared to benefit from it therapeutically, whilst other patients certainly become more manageable following it.

This role, however, was beginning to be questioned from within the hospital system itself. One doctor framed a different area of concern in relation to the quality of psychiatric treatment. Although a well-stocked arsenal of contemporary anti-psychotic drugs and tranquillisers were ready for use at Hospital Tranquillity, his fear was that medication prescribed on the wards was rarely reviewed throughout a patient's psychiatric 'career' and that consequently polypharmacology of obsolete prescriptions continued to be common practice. A senior psychiatrist agreed with this criticism but went further in expressing his concern that outpatients were frequently overmedicated and/or were receiving inappropriate medication.

Researcher:	Are you saying that people come into the psychiatric hospital with psychosis and are given very high dosages, but that they continue to get the same level when they are better?
AK:	Yes, because they are not being reassessed in their communities.
Researcher:	What are the repercussions of such high dosages?
AK:	Zombie-*ish* types of behaviour. Other effects as well. The illness role continues, you know, the illness behaviour is maintained. Other effects, like tardive (dyskinesia) which is more handicapping than the problem (illness). And those who really need medication don't get it – due to insight problems and rejection (of medication) by others.
Researcher:	It's a real paradox.
AK:	Yes, the ones that don't need it are given it....
Researcher:	How? By repeat prescriptions?

AK: By the clinics (rural clinics) and these people usually have very supportive families who get them the prescription. They (the family) are very helpful because they (the patient) are no bother. But people who are difficult, well people are scared of them and reject them, so they get no more treatment. And going to the clinic is difficult because of poverty and so on.

Given all these complex issues therefore it is somewhat strange that the 'non-compliance' of patients was not more fully accepted by ward staff in general as holding meanings other than that of a form of sickness behaviour. To do so, however, would no doubt mean a reorientation of the role of psychiatry as well as far-reaching logistical changes in service delivery. This would not only imply open dialogue with patients regarding the pros and cons of treatment but also a revision of treatment and how medication was prescribed, as well as reviewing the whole concept of consent to treatment in a realignment with the cultural context. Even if such a scenario were to be seen as an eventual goal, it would seem a remote one under the current circumstances.

Patient accounts clearly indicate that medication is viewed with anxiety and in some cases dread in the hospital setting, while in general it appears to be regarded as a necessary evil by staff. Compliant behaviour by the majority of inpatients in this respect does not imply equal acceptance, but is more likely to be a pragmatic response to a situation where great power is held by those in charge towards the issue of medication, rather than shared, even at a token level, with patients. Once discharged from this environment, neglect or rejection of prescribed medication by outpatients may well include a lack of comprehension of the benefits of medication in keeping psychiatric service users out of the institution. Yet this is also, and significantly so, an act of autonomy and defiance that would be forcibly repressed within the asylum system. Back within the institution, spirituality and mysticism, regardless of how this is visualised and articulated, becomes a culturally accepted means of expressing a transcendent vision of self that stands in opposition to a medicalised regime of depersonalisation and oppression.

7
Mad, wanton women and the feminine ideal

Unlike most visitors to the hospital, I was privileged in being allowed an almost unprecedented freedom to explore wards at my leisure. This was an irresistible research opportunity of which I took full advantage whenever I could. Thanks, therefore, to the generosity of the director I was able to make a more direct comparison of ward conditions than probably any other single individual at the hospital. Normally patients were not permitted access to other wards except under special circumstances, and this was particularly enforced in the case of women and male patients crossing the boundaries of the wards occupied by the opposite sex. Although such restrictions did not apply to staff, it was unusual for them to make regular forays out of their own domain, except on express business missions that did not encompass the motives or the methods of the inquisitive researcher.

'Open' and closed wards

One aspect that had fuelled my curiosity was to understand the complexities of the open ward system as it was practised at Hospital Tranquillity. The most interesting contrasts could be found through a comparison of the acute wards: Male and Female Wards 1. Although these wards were almost identical in layout they ran on very different lines and apparently autonomously, with an unclear relationship to hospital policy as I understood it.

While both wards contained a locked section for psychotic and generally unruly patients, the use of this facility appeared to be interpreted quite differently on the respective wards, but it took many months of observation and thought before an analysis emerged to sufficiently account for these differences. My first acquaintance with the locked-section phenomenon was that of Male Ward 1, which held the majority of patients at any given time, and as such was a very overcrowded and sordid environment. Facilities on the locked section in this ward reflected in part those of the open ward, yet were conspicuously older and more dilapidated. Thus the beds were old and rickety with poorer or even no bedding, which in any case consisted only of a plastic mattress, sheet and pillows. The walls were quite stained, especially near the bathroom with what looks like faecal matter, and were obviously less hygienic than the open ward. Altogether, the locked sections of Male Ward 1 and its female counterpart were unpleasant, odiferous and crowded, with several patients having to use the adjacent cramped and squalid bathroom. The following description taken from field notes illustrates the general environment of the locked section on Male Ward 1 on a typical day.

Field notes. Locked section, Male Ward 1

The MAs described the locked ward as being less crowded today but nonetheless patients were lying down in various places - on the mattresses or the floor. Some beds are without mattresses at all and patients lie on springs. On one bed with a mattress two patients are sleeping back to back. Under this bed a man sleeps on the bare floor, and next to him another. I notice the locked ward particularly today: the pale blue faded paint, the suspicious streaks of dirt and maybe faeces on the walls, especially near the toilet. The strong stench of excrement and the sheer barrenness of the environment. People sleep, as there is nothing else to do, one man sits staring into space. A deranged and giggling patient spots me and follows my movements through the bars, whatever he is saying completely incomprehensible.

The locked section on Male Ward 1 was marginally more squalid than that on Female Ward 1 where conditions were similar in terms of confinement under overcrowded conditions, while many patients of both sexes were evidently psychotic and often aggressive. This made the locked section on male and even female wards a particularly risky and highly disruptive environment to be in, as the following extract indicates.

Field notes. Female Ward 1.

By 8.10 (pm) the lights are turned out in the locked section, but people like Tuyah and Roslia (the rather sullen woman who spat at me) still stand at the bars talking and pacing around. A woman inside is screaming periodically. Earlier I saw her pulling, slapping and shouting at a prostrate patient.

Researcher:	There seems a lot of noise going on in there.
Nurse T:	Yes, she thinks someone is having sex with her. If you ask her, she'll tell you someone is trying to have sex with her.
Researcher:	Can the patients sleep with all that going on?
Nurse T:	Sometimes they are disturbed. Some patients will pull their sheets off, or pour water on them.
Researcher:	Pour water? That sounds pretty bad. What do you do?
Nurse T:	Tie them up maybe or separate them …. The problems at night-time are different from those in the day.

Though the locked sections on the male and female acute wards closely resembled each other in physical geography, they were run very differently. This reflected assumptions and stereotypes that related to conceptions of madness and idealised gender norms grounded in traditional attitudes. The locked sections of both wards were, however, a dominant feature of ward life, which most patients, would experience to a greater or lesser extent. The demarcation between open and locked sections on Male Ward 1 was clearly defined and there was little opportunity for close interaction between the two different categories of patient, short of the occasional chat or exchange of small items, such as cigarettes and snacks. Even during visiting hours male patients were not allowed out of the locked section to talk to their families in private, but contented themselves with sharing intimate moments, separated by bars, with the rest of the ward as involuntary witnesses. Virtually every man would have experience of the locked section in that for the vast majority this was their first experience of ward life following admission. As Peter, a young Dayak, first-admission patient, authoritatively informed me, 'everyone new is locked up'. Confinements like these could go on for days, and Teo and Chua, two disgruntled Chinese veterans and comrades agreed that, 'the worst thing on the ward is no freedom'. Once liberated from the locked section however, there was usually more scope for visits beyond the confines of the ward for recreation purposes.

The staff rationale behind the confinement of men lay in the need to prevent 'absconding' and 'escapes', for the assumption amongst most members of staff spoken to was that patients would certainly do so given the least opportunity. Escape prevention was therefore identified as a very important role in nursing supervision and methods of control were usually reframed as responsible measures demonstrating staff accountability. The language used by staff in relation to male patients and their freedom of movement was suggestive: the use of the term 'escape' in relation to men denoted a view of male patients as being very different from their female counterparts, who were deemed to be more accepting of their controlled environment. To contextualise this point both Jane Ussher (1991) and David Pilgrim (1988) argue that in the West male madness is deemed to be more dangerous than that of women's and consequently requires the use of a predominantly penal-type environment. This resonates with the view of staff at Tranquillity that male patient were more aggressive than women, as well as more independent and opportunistic. By contrast, although women were also subject to the careful vigilance of staff, this was based on an entirely different criterion, which served to perpetuate a view of femininity that stood in contrast with that denoting the masculine.

The relative liberty of male patients on the open section of the acute ward was not shared to anything approaching a similar degree with that of their female counterparts on Female Ward 1. Here the open/locked geography of the ward was subject to a different demarcation and flow of movement. Women on the acute ward were all confined to the ward and were not permitted to venture out unaccompanied at all. Nurses would escort small convoys of women patients to the occupational therapy department or to group exercise sessions, as well as to other forms of recreation, like the occasional ward party. Consequently, in an environment marked by enforced confinement of all patients, the demarcation between open and locked was less clearly drawn on the female wards. Yet of course certain women were relegated to the locked wards for disruptive behaviour of various sorts. They were primarily segregated from others during the night, for during the day it was quite normal practice to allow them to mingle with others on the open ward at selected times, or indeed for those at liberty on the open ward to choose to visit companions in the locked ward. The movement on the ward between these two distinct zones was therefore very fluid in the case of women patients, whilst the boundaries between the ward and access to the rest of hospital were carefully guarded by staff.

Male patients once liberated onto the open ward were much more likely to find themselves placed back in the locked section for antisocial behaviour. By contrast on Female Ward 1, while 'aggressive' women were uniformly disliked by staff in keeping with Chesler's (1996: 51) point, they were not solely confined to the locked ward but were free at times to mingle with others on the open section, which was of course not open but also locked. At Hospital Tranquillity, however, the boundaries between aggressive and placid behaviour in women were blurred through a general policy of confinement that made prisoners of female patients on the ward. The outcome was that violence by women patients could not be adequately curbed by similar strategies to those used with male patients, and other forms of control had to be created that were compatible with the idealised and helpless passivity of women (Redfield Jamison, 1996).

It appeared that women patients were regarded by nursing staff as requiring more supervision in general than their male counterparts, and reasons given for the strict confinement of women were commensurate with this assumption. Women patients were viewed in terms of vulnerability and social responsibility, and their sexuality was seen to be a commodity that needed to be controlled by staff (McGinty, 1996).

The control of women's sexuality at Tranquillity crosses many religious and cultural traditions in keeping with the nation's multifaith and multicultural conventions. Consequently the drive to keep women patients confined to their wards, while men are permitted to wander afield, is not so far removed from the practices of the Iban or Wana of Central Sulawesi. In both ethnic groups, women are expected to remain close to home, while men are free to travel beyond the community boundaries. Moreover, for the Wana the surrounding forest is seen as essentially a masculine domain. It is completely out of bounds to women to the extent that the threat of rape of kinswomen disobedient in this regard is used to enforce the message of the 'inappropriateness of women venturing into the forest, the site of men's activities...' (Monnig Atkinson, 1990: 85). Mirroring this situation, staff at the hospital were equally dedicated towards preventing women in their care from falling prey to sexual attacks in the areas beyond the confines of the women's wards.

Additionally, the sequestering of women patients at Tranquillity bears many of the hallmarks of a Judaeo-Christian-Islamic heritage, preoccupied with women's chastity in keeping with their dispossession of an autonomous self. Equally then, and in direct comparison with Italian psychiatric hospitals in the 1960s and 1970s, women patients at Tranquillity were strongly identified within their biological roles (Cogliati et al., 1988: 101). Significantly, the majority of women patients on Female Ward 1 were of childbearing age and accordingly their liberty was habitually circumscribed, reminiscent of Elaine Showalter's description of nineteenth-century institutional care.

> For as the Victorian asylums became more overtly benign, protective and custodial it also became an environment grotesquely like the one in which women normally functioned e.g. strict chaperonage, restraint of movement

and limited occupation, enforced sexlessness and constant subjugation to authority (Showalter, 1981: 321).

At Tranquillity, the position of young fertile women patients stood in some contrast to the position of obviously post-menopausal elderly counterparts on the chronic wards, who were more likely to be permitted greater latitude to wander the adjacent corridors, provided they did not go beyond the hospital boundaries. Furthermore, by subsuming the concepts of gender/sexuality/fertility these then become subject to further refinement on the grounds of class distinctions, as such constraints applied specifically to women on the 'public' wards. Pre-menopausal women on the private wards were 'supervised' by staff, but this was more likely to be restricted to judicious chaperonage, rather than to literal confinement. Although equally subject to patriarchal definitions of the 'feminine' this was applied according to more genteel standards in keeping with the social status of the bourgeoisie. Regardless of class however, as Cogliati et al. (1988: 101) note, 'women of all classes' are essentially 'reduced to being only bodies'. In this vein Phyllis Chesler (1996) goes on to argue that women generically in asylum care have traditionally been subject to very close supervision, in which the notion of women's essential and childlike dependency on psuedo-professional parenting is reinforced through control and the punishment of 'wayward' behaviour.

The gender of women with psychiatric histories at Tranquillity can therefore be interpreted as subject to an analysis of binary opposition, whereby women with mental illnesses were seen as virginal, childlike and potentially vulnerable victims of unscrupulous men (Beasley, 1999). This can be read as an identification of women patients with the mad woman in her innocent Ophelia mode (Kromm, 1994). On the other hand, as typified by the Bertha Rochester image from Charlotte Bronte's Jane Eyre, women patients can be simultaneously seen as predatory and promiscuous, inclined to solicit sexual intercourse without discrimination.

Jenny on Female Ward 1 exemplified the concept of the simple and deceived innocent. This was a quiet individual with mild learning disabilities who had been recently readmitted onto the ward ostensibly due to a pregnancy, her second by the same man. She was instantly categorised by staff as a 'rape victim' or at least as a victim of seduction by a wily opportunist, which was seen as much the same situation. Jenny herself seemed pleased about her pregnancy and referred to her impregnator as 'her boyfriend', this being passed off as a sign of her naiveté and inability to care for herself. Because Jenny was seen as a particularly vulnerable woman staff decided that she would not be allowed to keep her baby, and sought to 'protect' her by arranging for a non-voluntary sterilisation at the general hospital, and the enforced adoption of her baby through the welfare services.

The rationale behind such close supervision of women patients conforms to the notion of women as essentially wanton, weak and corrupt, to paraphrase Cogliati et al. (1988), as the following section of interview indicates:

Researcher:	So you think they (women patients) may be abused if they go out?
Nurse L:	Maybe … We have a deaf one, maybe she has – and some like it. Maybe their trade and they go back to it!

While on a different occasion another nurse confirmed this view in the following way: 'women can be raped, men can't, but some women even go out and invite it!' Thus the relationship between madness and unbridled sexuality was one that is embedded in traditional stereotypes of women's madness as being untrammelled, uncontainable and subversive in its threat to a social fabric that relies on the 'good' woman's basic chastity and frigidity as tokens of female sanity and gender conformity.

Accordingly, the open ward system on Female Ward 1 was criticised by some members of staff on the grounds that this enabled women patients to enjoy a dangerous freedom. Yet the complex nuances behind this use of an 'open' but actually locked system was sufficiently incongruous for some members of staff to try and justify it to interested listeners, such as myself:

Field notes. Female Ward 1.

It's the end of the day. I am tired and want to leave but first have to find a nurse to let me out of the ward. As she does so for some reason Nurse S feels the need to explain about the locked grill gate.

Nurse S:	Years ago it (gate) was open … but a patient had a baby.
Researcher:	You mean she got pregnant by another patient?
Nurse S:	Yes – relations with another patient. It was a baby girl, delivered in XGH (XGeneral Hospital). I think she was adopted …. The hospital was short-handed then.
Researcher:	Is the ward short-handed now?
Nurse S:	Not so much.

The inference drawn therefore was that even if the public were unable to 'abuse' women patients, they were still vulnerable to the attentions of male patients who might impregnate them, as had already happened. In actual fact despite this allegation being repeated to me by two different parties, this event was denied by other long-serving nurses familiar with the female wards. In addition, I found no real evidence that this event really took place, and suggest that it may have formed a useful piece of staff mythology that worked against the free movement of female patients.

In either case women, whether reluctant or active participants in heterosexual encounters, were seen in terms of biological functions that were subject to moral codes and therefore in need of close surveillance (Cogliati, et al., 1988; Ussher, 1991). Consequently strict sexual segregation at Tranquillity was viewed not as social control but more as a means of protection of women in custodial care. This reflects measures in contemporary Britain where isolation of sexually 'disinhibited' women away from male 'exploitation' is defended as a safety measure (Mental Health Act Commission, 1997: 10; SNMAC, 1999). Furthermore this is commensurate with Gittins' rather more sympathetic interpretation of similar procedures in pre-Second World War England, in that sexually segregated areas for women could be viewed as a place of sanctuary rather than oppression in that they

> Provided shelter, protection and 'asylum' from an outside world in which violence and abuse by men could be, and frequently had been terrifying (Gittins, 1998: 127).

On the female wards at Tranquillity, however, notions relating to the passivity, vulnerability and chastity of women were reinforced as feminine ideals that counterbalanced the view of women patients as sexually predatory and therefore equally in need of segregation from men. In reality the consequence was that this policy tended to generate behaviour that subsequently justified its continuation. On Female Ward 1, women patients often responded to youthful visiting male doctors with a lusty lack of inhibition that one would normally associate with a certain type of juvenile, machismo, in-group behaviour overtly designed to sexually humiliate women. Ironically in the course of their duties these mortified young doctors found themselves placed in the inverted and ignominious position of becoming objects of sexual gratification to a whooping, bar-rattling, audience of harpies shooting lewd remarks in their direction.

Sexual disinhibition and mental illness in women has historically been viewed as constituting a causal relationship, with the concept of 'nymphomania' (with the implicit assumption of promiscuity and masturbatory excesses), prescribed by unseemly energy in behaviour and speech, together with the rejection of feminine social graces, and a lack of shyness. Such activities, uncharacteristic of rigid definitions of the feminine in nineteenth century Europe, did not necessarily have to be accompanied by overt sexual activity to be labelled the hallmark of nymphomania (Goldberg, 1999). Goldberg goes on informs us that the cure for such subversion in women was to attempt to quench their heightened appetites through a range of methods, including insipid diets, purges, cold water and mechanical restraints, such as the straitjacket or solitary confinement. By contrast, sexual subversion in men, in the form of masturbation was viewed as rendering men furtive, devoid of masculine energy and purpose. Thus, the cure for such lack of characteristic potency was the reverse to that of women in terms of dietary considerations and the partaking of wholesome exercise (Goldberg, 1999).

Such descriptions retain the air of anachronistic curiosities of little relevance to modern psychiatric care; nevertheless, some evocative resonances remain detectable down the corridors of institutional care historically. For example, male patients at Tranquillity, whether by accident or design, do benefit from greater freedom and often a wider choice of diet compared to their female counterparts. The hospital football pitch is effectively a recreation for male patients, as is the badminton court. Women, as we will see, have other recreational outlets provided to them, where, as Chesler (1994: xix) comments, they are encouraged to make a necessary adjustment to the 'feminine' role as 'the measure of female morality, mental health, and psychiatric progress'.

As Showalter (1981: 320) points out in comparison with Chesler's observation, removed from the social constraints of normal society women psychiatric patients are liberated to express themselves in rowdy behaviour which challenges the female stereotype '… that women should be quiet, virtuous and immobile'. This, however, did not serve to overturn notions of gender norms prevalent among staff, but instead mandated that these norms should be reinforced, if necessary by punitive measures. Commensurate with this was the practice of tying patients to beds with cotton restraints that was still widely used at Hospital Tranquillity, and particularly on women of all ages, including the infirm elderly. It was therefore quite common to find restraints used on elderly and infirm individuals of both sexes as a means of ensuring immobility that was overtly seen by staff as a risk management procedure to prevent injury or inappropriate movements, particularly in the case of impending senility. In this respect both the infirm elderly and pre-menopausal women were seen as occupying a similar category of being fundamentally irresponsible: a danger to themselves, yet essentially impotent for which physical control was the best cure.

The use of restraints on women is by no means unique to this hospital, however, and was noted to be a facet of nineteenth century asylum care in both Europe and the notorious institutions in America (Geller and Harris, 1994). It was also a feature to some extent in Italian psychiatric practice in the recent past, in keeping with the hostile professional attitude towards women in asylum care (Cogliati et al., 1988: 99). At Tranquillity restraints were used on women generally for 'behavioural problems', such as acts of disobedience and aggression. The whole notion that physical passivity was normal for women, and that confinement was an appropriate management technique compatible with gender difference, was one that was seen to be powerfully reinforced on the female wards (Showalter, 1981).

The following dialogue, which took place with the friendly if inarticulate Wei Hua and her rather taciturn companion Noor from Female Ward 1, offers a perspective of how confinement was experienced and understood by women patients.

Researcher:	[To Noor] Have you been in the locked section?
[General laughter]	
Noor:	Of course! We've all been in the locked section.
Wei Hua:	I go to locked section!
Researcher:	What was it like?
Noor:	Bad. There are bad smells from the jamban (latrines), when you sleep, when you eat, very bad.
Researcher:	Why do people go to the locked section?
Noor:	When you scream, when you shout, when you behave badly you go to the locked section. When you fight – fighting for freedom you are restrained. (Gloomily) I was restrained yesterday.
Researcher:	Why was that?
Noor:	I put my gold ...[indicates neck and searches for word] pendant down the jamban. They tied my hands [puts her arms crucifixion-style] and tied. My hands hurt.
[She shows me faint bruises on her wrists].	
Researcher:	How did you feel about that?
Noor:	I cried, I felt so bad. 2 hours on the bed. Legs are tied very tight. That is not the law to restrain when they are sick.

	Knocked my head on the bed, nurse Sister X. Very harsh treatment.
Wei Hua:	(Vaguely) My sister's baby, it screamed and screamed and she put it ... tied it in... a sarong and put it in the bed and gave the baby her susu (milk/breast)... and the baby... (tails off)

For Noor confinement on the locked ward was a deeply disagreeable physical experience, but being tied to her bed was, she conveyed, worse in being a psychological and physical assault of the deepest degradation. Understandably, Noor showed deep suspicion and resentment of the nursing staff in general, and regarded many of their actions towards patients as being forms of punishment for resistance. Wei Hua however seemed to take a different stance, as indicated by her interjection, which seemed rather bizarre and unconnected with the topic discussed, although she was at the time listening attentively to my conversation with Noor. Whereas Noor viewed restraints as no less than utterly brutal, Wei Hua appeared to draw an association between confinement and protective containment and parental care. This to some extent reflects Chesler's analysis of psychiatric nurses acting out the role of *ersatz* authoritative and smothering/mothering figures: in that the bondage of women was apparently seen by Wei Hua as in some way analogous to the swaddling of infants by loving figures of authority, and therefore forgivable if misconceived (Chesler, 1972; Chesler, 1996).

It becomes apparent that the disciplinary nature of forcibly immobilising women – through the general policy of the locked section and the discretionary practice of using restraints – is in effect a crude method of reinforcing patriarchal definitions of gender, as well as acting as a means of social control. Just as the suppression of their heterosexuality gives rise to exaggerated displays of sexual consciousness by women, as well as frustration on the wards, the efforts to enforce passivity and modesty on women served to emphasise their sexual identity as primarily that of objects of male sexual gratification. Even this role, however, could not be gratified due to their status as psychiatric patients, and consequently the women held this objectivised, sexualised self in indefinite suspension. Unsurprisingly therefore expressions of sexuality became an introverted preoccupation with grooming for a forbidden role, while narcissistic occupations were equally encouraged as appropriate leisure pursuits on the female wards.

Gender and recreation

Traditionally male patients have been regarded as naturally and obviously benefiting from outdoor activities, and at Tranquillity men on both the acute and chronic wards could look forward to leisure activities beyond the confines of their ward; playing football at the entrance to the hospital, for instance (Gittins, 1998: 127). A recently installed badminton area on Male Ward 1 stood testimony to the notion that expenditure of physical energy was a normal and appropriate masculine pursuit. This clearly was not regarded as important for women however, whose leisure pursuits by contrast almost solely took place in the ward environment itself and here gender-appropriate recreation was encouraged. On Female Ward 1 women were encouraged to listen to pop music, or endlessly leaf through women's magazines liberally littered with advertisements for beauty aids for the lightening of dark skins. Alternatively on Friday mornings for the 'chronic' patients on Female Ward 2 there were newly implemented make-up sessions to look forward to.

In her study of the American beauty culture, Kathrin Perutz (1971) draws attention to the use of cosmetics as a therapeutic strategy for women psychiatric service users, claiming that 'beauty therapy' is now a common addition in the psychiatrist's arsenal. The aim is to achieve 'normalcy', interpreted by Perutz (1971: 192) as meaning uncontested heterosexuality and a self-absorbed attention to grooming. In this analysis women are obliged to project a socially accepted, normative appearance as a necessary condition for uniting an otherwise fragmented, self-alienated psyche. The goal is to achieve better social relations specifically with the other sex and thereby, on the surface at least, demonstrate social conformity and good adjustment to the female role in society. The underlying assumption being that such women are otherwise physically and socially unattractive, desexualised or worse still, probably lesbian, and thus effectively socially dead.

This analysis of the power of cosmetics, and all such associated narcissistic behaviour, is reminiscent of the observation by Rowett and Vaughan (1981: 137) in their study of women offenders in the UK, where inmates are regarded as making clear progress towards 'recovery' by the controlling authorities if they adopt overtly feminine interests that are compatible with gender normative behaviour.

Unsurprisingly therefore the adoption of beauty sessions was considered by the nurses to be a highly popular innovation for patients, although the recreational aspects were emphasised rather more than a professional parade of presumed therapeutic benefits. Used cosmetics and other feminine props were generously donated by staff for these dressing-up sessions, in which even the most confused patients appeared to join in. Most female patients could be found applying make-up with enormous care and devotion to detail, showing a rare and often exceptional concentration. In contrast to the seriousness with which these women took these activities many of the nurses appeared to find these sessions a source of entertainment and sat in groups looking on, commenting and laughing at the antics and pretensions so openly displayed. Yet as a spectator myself, the nurses' amusement did not seem to me to be just callous mirth, but a reaction to a fundamental discomfort with the proceedings, as certainly there was something touching but macabre about the spectacle as this extract from field notes conveys.

Field notes. Female Ward 2

Mae, a mentally disabled and rather alarming woman who carries the battered, broken-nosed face of a convict, applies a heavy dusting of talcum powder to her face. On top she adds two large rings of lipstick onto her cheeks and also applies this to her lips, grinning with pleasure and showing half-rotted teeth. Later she works and reworks the palette of her face with bright pink rouge and so on, until she looks quite frightful. At the next table the nurses keep an eye on the patients, having a bit of a giggle at the mess they are making. Margot applies makeup carefully and with dignity: green eye shadow, face powder, muted lipstick. I have rarely seen her look so nice. I compliment her and she laughs. 'No, no - I look like the devil!' she says in her half-amused, half-mournful self-depreciating way. A serious, elderly stooped patient stolidly paints the face of another elderly patient incompetently but caringly. Another has painted her face into a travesty of a Japanese geisha, all white powder and bright pink cheeks and eyes, with dark eyebrows and red lipstick. She scowls at me watching her.

As Perutz argues, these sessions seemed to act as a tangible reminder to women patients of their sex, as well as some of the expectations attached to gender, with concern for appearance, narcissism and decorum being inculcated in women from an early age. Furthermore, female staff epitomised through scrupulous dress and careful grooming the ideals of feminine beauty which women patients could aspire to but never attain. However, although the end result often looked like a travesty of femininity, the chance to recreate oneself, and the concentration required in creating these geisha-like masks were undeniable, remarkable and unnerving in this stultifying environment. On Female Ward 1 if a woman attempted against the odds to overcome the desexualisation of generic, regimented, unkempt patient-hood through acts of self-ornamentation staff would reinforce this through such verbalised approved as, *'cantik!'* (lovely) you look pretty today', a clear message of approval by those who normally suppressed signs of asserted individually.

Pictures of predominantly white glamour models and a faded photograph of fetching blonde Aryan children also reminded women patients that the accepted hallmarks of beauty were seen as belonging primarily to the fair-skinned races. As one nurse commented to me with bland irony, 'all white people are beautiful'. Consequently, and to my dismay, I was regularly courted with compliments by patients on my otherwise unremarkable Caucasian features. Further, as towards a precocious and lovable child, I was regularly patted and petted with the occasional lesbian overture thrown in to boot. On one memorable occasion I received a long love letter from a woman starting with the words, 'to the first *orang puteh* (white person) I have loved ….' from which it was apparent that my appearance alone had managed to conjure up fantasies for my admirer that were otherwise devoid of reality and could not therefore be realised. This was more than partially expected from my admirer, who as befits the besotted, expected to enjoy an unrequited love and to adore only from afar.

The lesbian alternative

In the strict confines of an environment where sexuality was both highlighted and denied by the system it was of course predictable that patients would seek gratification through homosexual alliances. Most of my information on this subject was gathered from observation and interviews with female patient respondents. By comparison, although some male patients had clearly adopted a 'gay' identity, or, as in the case of Miss Hui Ling, a female identity, these men practically never alluded to this aspect of their lives. Equally male staff were unwilling to discuss this directly, although some did admit that homosexual acts regularly took place on the wards, but that these were somehow 'prevented', yet how exactly was not explained. The reluctance to discuss this topic is matches general social attitudes towards gay lifestyles in Malaysia, which are informally practised and have given rise to an active street industry of cross-gender rent-boys, but are rarely discussed or socially acknowledged (Ashencaen Crabtree and Baba, 2001).

On the female wards, my investigations into lesbian relationships were treated with less circumspection than on the male wards. This was probably because although equally proscribed in Islam, in Malaysia lesbianism is barely recognised as a legitimate phenomenon (Ashencaen Crabtree and Ismail Baba, 2001). It therefore has no accepted social reality and does not pose as threat to cultural values in the same way as the male gay lifestyle. In opposition to this view Wazir Jahan Karim asserts that, in fact, normative sex roles are not as strictly demarcated as they are in the West and that some Asian women enjoy greater liberty to explore their sexuality, as indeed do their male counterparts.

> Numerous Southeast Asian cultures allow both men and women to explore their sexual differences freely, without inhibition and without shifting the natural attributes which both sexes have to offer one another (Karim, 1995: 36).

My research findings, however, differed widely from Karim's emancipated statement, in that at Tranquillity a conventional attitude of disapproval and discrimination was applied to women who did not conform to behaviours that in the West would be seen as gender normative. The resulting reactions and attitudes of those in authority towards these breaches were again similar to that which traditionally one would expect in a Western context, as described by Cogliati et al. (1988: 99) and additionally Chesler (1996), where lesbian conduct is subject to earnest repression in institutional care. Consequently, not all nurses admitted that lesbian relationships did exist on the wards and some categorically denied this even in the face of evidence. On one occasion I saw two inseparable women patients cuddling intimately but playfully in bed, the nurse I was with looked on stonily without interference, except to say to me eventually with disgust and resignation, 'Look at them – just like animals!'. What I found particularly interesting was this was the same nurse who had earlier told me that lesbian relations did not take place on this ward; clearly this represented more than just a problem of definition for this person. On another occasion a nurse attempted to be particularly helpful by pointing out an alleged lesbian couple and then paraded them in front of me as a supremely ridiculous example of a butch/femme stereotype. Fortunately, despite staff reluctance I was able to discuss these events with women patients with more success, such as in the following conversation with Soo Mei and friends.

Soo Mei: I love my friends ...[passionately grabs my hand]. But I don't like some ... We were in bed .... And I was like this - in the

> middle … and she touched my…susu (meaning breast) … and I said 'no' and … [gesture of hitting out]. Now she is afraid of me.

Researcher: What do you mean 'in the middle'?

Soo Mei: Like this …

[Draws a picture of 2 beds pushed together with three people lying in it]

Researcher: And that happened here? On the ward?

Aini: Yes, here!

Soo Mei: Yes, I scolded her!

[Points out one of the patients walking near us]. I don't like her.

[Tuyah comes up and joins us but is feeling withdrawn and unresponsive today]

Researcher: Do you have a boyfriend at home Soo Mei?

Soo Mei: Yes, I had a boyfriend one time but he wanted -

Aini: Sexuality!

Soo Mei: Make love. So I said 'No! do not… do not…' [lost for words]

Researcher: Tidak masuk (do not enter/penetrate)?

Soo Mei: Tidak masuk. I do not look like a …. soft … soft lady.

Aini: A soft lady, a gentle lady! You are a tomboy!

('Tomboy' carries certain connotations)

Soo Mei: I'm not a tomboy!

Aini: [To Tuyah laughing] A lesbian! A lesbian!

[Tuyah nods sullenly].

Although Soo Mei actively sought sexual gratification, she refused to be preyed upon by others and felt able to reject, if necessary violently, those lesbian advances that did not appeal to her. Although evidently ambivalent about being herself publicly labelled a lesbian, in her own forthright, assertive way Soo Mei projected a positive image of the lesbian alternative to the enforced chastity and sexual inertia of the sequestered and ideal female hetero-orientated patient. The 'tomboy' reference in its implication that lesbian sexuality emulates the active male role was one that Soo Mei shunned due probably to stigma, but also demonstrated through the adoption of boyish, uninhibited mannerisms and her smart masculine dress.

Aini, as a Muslim however, could not bring herself to condone lesbian behaviour and in fact indicated that an element of sexual violence permeated the ward system, in which she implicated both patients and staff.

Researcher: Why does she do that?

Aini: [Looking cautiously back to the nurses station] I don't know.

	(The patients) show their body - no shame. That is an issue of morality. The nurses come to take off my long pants, I think it's sexual – you say sexual? They touch [indicates breasts].
Researcher:	The patients show their bodies?
Aini:	I don't want that - that is lesbian and bad thing by God. Lesbian behaviour ... [Roughly grasps her breasts and vulva in clawed hands]. Some here - not a lot, during the day-time when I am bathing ... people are naked, bodies open to all.
Researcher:	What do the nurses do if that happens?
Aini:	The nurses scold but nothing. I pushed her off. The nurses locked her up and the nurses said something bad about me - I didn't hear them but heard them mumbling something.

My understanding was that Aini was evidently describing an attempted sexual assault by a fellow patient, although it was unclear to me how common such events were on the ward. Nonetheless Aini's point stands: that sexual assaults were not necessarily recognised by staff, who appear to equally condemn sexual assaults and consensual sex amongst women. Given the accounts by patient and staff participants the attitude of nurses towards anyone engaged in or suspected of lesbian behaviour was highly condemnatory. Under ideal circumstances the lesbian alternative could represent a way of subverting the 'cloistered' existence of women on the ward through sexual gratification that precluded the physically real or implied male presence (Mohanty, 1991). In opposition to this strategy, the ward environment was one where women patients in general were frequently obliged to adopt the posture of passive objects which could be publicly stripped of their clothing, and exposed in their nakedness to the voyeurism and even brutality of others. At the same time, through their condemnation of lesbian conduct but their general complacency towards sexual assaults on women patients by other women, nurses, as Chesler (1996) points out, fail to adequately protect women in their care. Regardless of the nature of any potential sexual contact, whether this was construed as heterosexual or lesbian, coerced or freely sought, women psychiatric patients at Tranquillity were regarded as morally culpable, sexually indiscriminate and therefore in need of surveillance and heavy measures of 'sociosexual' control that were essentially deeply stigmatising and punitive (Showalter, 1981).

8
Strategies of containment on the ward

In Malaysia, racial and ethnic questions normally revolve around the safer topic of multicultural celebration rather than dissonance: unity rather than fragmentation, overall progress rather than racial discrimination. Particularly so, as memories of the race riots of 1969 where hundreds of people were slaughtered have dimmed but not disappeared from mind. These events are unlikely to be repeated, in view of the development of affirmative action policies towards the *bumiputera* (Ashencaen Crabtree, 1999bc; Baba et al., 2010). In the meantime, open dialogue on racially sensitive issues is suppressed and the privileges rendered to the status of the *bumiputera* to-date remain inviolable.

As mentioned in Chapter One, affirmative policies dictate where non-*bumiputera* may buy land, leading to a ghettoising effect of ethnic concentration in neighbourhoods, and duly inflated property prices in these localities. Quotas for tertiary education and civil service employment discriminate against predominantly Chinese and Indian citizens as well as any other category not falling into the privileged First Citizen status of the *bumiputera*. Such disenfranchising but popular policies cost the country a good deal in terms of finances and human resources, but are unlikely to be reversed in the foreseeable future due to the political threat of a sunk revenue of votes at the polls.

The relationship between ethnicity, social assimilation and psychiatric morbidity is therefore not one that is easily explored. Accordingly, Rostom and Lee (1996), both Malaysian-born academics, conclude their report on psychiatric institutions in Peninsular Malaysia by applauding the way services meet the cultural needs of patients through observing 'cultural, spiritual, religious and dietary' norms. To some extent, this occurs at Tranquillity as well through the celebration of local, ethnic festivities on the wards. A multicultural patient population notwithstanding, one of the more conspicuous aspects of life at Tranquillity is the high numbers of Chinese patients of both sexes on virtually every ward. This predominance can hardly be ignored and hospital records confirm that Chinese patients form the overall majority of patients.

In order to put this into some sort of context however, early on in the fieldwork process figures relating to ethnic breakdown were compared with Hospital Bukit Padang in Sabah (a small hospital of 302 beds) and Hospital Bahagia in the State of Perak (an enormous hospital offering approximately 2,600 beds). These were reviewed in relation to the official population census of the States and the results duly compared (Department of Statistics, 1991) (Appendix I, Table 4). Based on these variables it could be seen that at Tranquillity figures for multiply-admitted Chinese patients in 1998 of both sexes stood at 43% of the overall hospital population, and commensurately first-admission patients stood at 34%. In 2006, the overall population of Chinese inpatients stood at 49%, compared to a combined Dayak inpatient population of 50%. Compare this to the Chinese general population in 1998 where the Census records their presence at standing at 28% of the overall population. It should also be noted that the hospital population as a whole supports a high concentration of Chinese patients amongst the 'chronic' population, as a typical 'snapshot' of demographics of four wards indicates.

Table 1
Hospital Tranquillity – Ethnic breakdown and inpatients (2000)

Acute Ward	Chronic Ward	Ethnic breakdown
Male Ward 1		Chinese: 17 Malay: 5 Dayak: 11 Other: 1
Female Ward 1		Chinese: 18 Malay: 7 Dayak: 6
	Male Ward 2	Chinese: 26 Malay: 2 Dayak: 4 Other: 1
	Female Ward 2	Chinese: 34 Malay: 1 Dayak: 7

The Perak and Sabah hospitals suggest that a similar scenario was played out to that of Hospital Tranquillity at the turn of the millennium.

Here, despite the contrast in population percentages, such as that in Perak, the Chinese population was roughly half the number of Malays, whereas in Sabah the opposite situation held: Chinese still outnumbered Malay patients considerably by a high ratio. In Perak Chinese patients formed 29.4% of the population, yet showed a 38% presence in the psychiatric hospital. Furthermore, despite a small National and State presence of 9.5%, Indian patients in Perak were equally over-represented, standing at 17% of the patient population. In Sabah the Chinese civil population has been relatively high at 15.6%, but the corresponding patient population has stood over twice that level at 34%. By 2009, on a return visit to Tranquility, I noted that the high number of Chinese patients continued to be a notable feature of the patient population, which was not surprising given the large number of chronic patients whose permanent residence was effectively long stay hospitalization.

The preponderance of long-stay Chinese patients of both sexes in a contemporary Malaysian psychiatric hospital offers some useful insights in relation to similar findings of asylum care and ethnic breakdown in colonial Malaya, where migrant workers dominated the patient population (Tan and Wagner, 1971; Jin Inn Teoh, 1971). Similarly, the low numbers of locals in psychiatric resources during the colonial period has been reflected in modern day Hospital Tranquillity, where an outstanding feature is the under-representation of Dayak patients. Yet in terms of population percentages in East Malaysia they collectively represent a large majority. However, anomalies exist: the indigenous Borneo Melanau are categorised according to religious rather than ethnic background, as are the Orang Asli of the Peninsula. Specifically, those Melanau who have converted to Islam are accorded the honorary status of *Malay*, whereas Melanau Christians remain in their original category of *Dayak*. The significance of this noteworthy fact carries resonance in terms of camouflaging ethnic representation in government statistics, although Melanaus are very much a minority ethnic group in any case.

In total, these findings are suggestive and resonate strongly with the views of Nazroo (1997) and Rack (1982) in suggesting that migration issues appear to play a significant role with regards to the mental health of ethnic groups. In accordance with this, despite acculturation, succeeding generations apparently remain susceptible to the diagnosis of mental illness, particularly when compounded by the oppression of institutional racism in contemporary society (Barnes and Bowl, 2001; Fernando *et al.*, 1988).

Moral containment of patients and ethnic typecasting

Intrigued by this situation, I spent a good deal of time questioning staff at Tranquillity on these discrepancies. The problems teasing out these issues were compounded by the fact that two important areas of stigma, racial discrimination and mental illness, directly overlapped in the case of Chinese patients. This was therefore a very sensitive threshold to cross, especially for Chinese members of staff, who were understandably reluctant to discuss this openly, or otherwise sought to distance themselves personally from any negative associations that might accompany ethnic predominance.

If Chinese staff were reluctant to speak, staff from other ethnic backgrounds were usually more willing to oblige, openly airing their views of ethnic predominance through personal interpretation of cultural and racial difference that served to highlight assumptions and indeed prejudices on ethnic grounds. The situation on *Bunga Raya* ward provides a useful illustration, in that here the ethnic breakdown was reversed and permanent residents were more likely to be of Iban and Malay origin rather than Chinese or Bidayuh. Explanations for this were again based on the mythology of ethnic difference and related to the 'impulsive, violent, lacking self-control – no thought for the consequences' behaviour of Iban patients, for example, as described by a senior Chinese medical assistant. This description, however, fits the hyper-masculinised warrior image that is popularly associated with this particular ethnic group and which, to some extent, is still promoted with pride. Whereas, the MA went on to say that the Chinese by contrast have a lot of 'self-control', but were regarded in general as docile (carrying overtones of demasculinised passivity and impotence) and predisposed to schizophrenia. On one of the chronic wards, a Dayak medical assistant had this to say on the subject of Chinese attitudes towards mental illness:

> They don't like mental illness in the family, it's seen as bad luck, so they (patients) are dumped here, but with Malay families even if someone is very very ill they still visit. Chinese people are very superstitious.

The Chinese family was often portrayed in staff and patient accounts as being highly competitive, exceedingly hardworking, as well as insular, family and clan orientated. In addition they were also depicted as mercenary and potentially pitiless with unproductive members of family, especially if these are stricken with mental illness (Ashencaen Crabtree, 1999b, Chen, 1995).

Thus, the old stereotype of the Chinese migrant entrepreneur, ruthlessly exploiting any avenue for gain, was revived in these accounts to be deplored, disliked and resented all over again by those from other ethnic heritages. The additional spice for these speakers, however, was that the migrants carried the seed of their own downfall in the shape of a predisposition to madness and in a particularly feminised form.

For certain members of staff, perhaps those more likely to attempt to put forward a balanced point of view, the power of stigma was proffered as a reason for the high numbers of patients. This was the explanation more likely to be put forward by Chinese staff members, following from that given by a high-ranking Chinese hospital administrator.

> *The Chinese believe in a genetic disposition. This tends to damn the whole family, including siblings, who may have a higher difficulty in finding a spouse, lah. Another reason is that the patient is not to blame but they may have done something terrible in a past life. And it may not be what they have done but an ancestor. The Chinese believe in cause and effect – karma, bad stock, but (this is) also a question of morality. The Chinese consider them (psychiatric patients) to be a shame and must be hidden, otherwise brothers and sisters affected. Madness is incurable … education won't help because they still believe it comes from past wrongs. The only thing we can do is to educate them into distinguishing between milder and more severe illnesses.*

This explanation furthermore is compatible with that put forward by Rack, who points out that where there is no obvious external cause for mental illness it is natural to ascribe a causation to something 'in the blood' (Rack, 1982: 173). This also provides a good reason for social rejection of the afflicted and stigmatised, and serves in turn to give a plausible account for the high numbers of chronic patients at Tranquillity (Yee and Au, 1997), in agreement with Arthur Kleinman:

> … stigma associated with categorizing individuals as mad in Chinese culture is more severe than that in the West, since the stigma attaches not just to the family member, but to the family as a whole (Kleinman, 1988b: 49).

Sometimes non-Chinese staff members adopted the explanation of stigma overtly but used this as a convenient vehicle to articulate their own prejudice, as in the case of a Dayak medical assistant in discussing qualities reputed to be typically Chinese.

> *Stigma! Chinese people don't want someone ill like this living with them. They*

don't want anyone to know, so they send them here. We natives show more love
for our relatives and keep them with us, but not the Chinese .... Some do visit
the patients here but they are more than Chinese – they are Christians and they
must love others... Most Chinese ... [dismissive hand gesture] they are too busy
making money.

A Dayak nurse on another occasion pointed out a Chinese patient on
Female Ward 1 to illustrate a point regarding the propensity of the Chinese
to mental illness and to desertion by their families:

You see her. You should visit her house [disgusted expression]. They have a big
statue in the house, maybe Buddha, and (joss) sticks everywhere, it is eerie, is that
how you say it? Probably that is what made her ill, her and her sister - they are
both here. The parents seem to want them to stay here, they don't take them home.

Here then the issue of religion is used to illustrate the 'Otherness' of
the Chinese. Wherein the natural avariciousness and ambition seen to be
typical of Chinese people by some members of staff, are redeemed through,
for instance, Christian principle, but adherence to their own set of values
(in this case Buddhism) is both alien, alienating and of dubious morality.
Chinese values for these informants are often sharply contrasted with
the apparent and much lauded 'tolerance' of Dayak and Malay families,
this being a commonly held assumption in the hospital, supported to some
extent in other research studies of Chinese, Malay and Indian families
(Bentelspacher *et al.*, 1994). Although interestingly a similar study
conducted by Wintersteen *et al.* (1997) did not find any conclusive evidence
of this cultural trend. Nonetheless at Tranquillity the belief persists, and is
particularly held by staff from other ethnic groups, that Chinese families are
more neglectful of relatives with mental illnesses than other ethnic groups.
This view underscores racist stereotypes, which do little to challenge the
accepted view that Chinese patients are often the helpless victims of their
own cultural cul-de-sac, thereby avoiding placing the phenomenon in the
wider context of social accommodation and assimilation of ethnic diversity
(Ashencaen Crabtree, 2001).
Staff accounts tended to confirm a general notion that the Chinese as
an ethnic group were therefore predisposed and susceptible to developing
psychiatric problems. An interesting comparison can once again be drawn
between Malaysia and Britain in exploring the circumstances of migration
and the preponderance of mental illness in the descendents. By contrast,
racist beliefs concerning the overrepresentation of African-Caribbean
people in psychiatric care are reversed in the Malaysian context (Fernando,

1995; Kleinman, 1988b). Ironically, a study of 'Bajan-Brits': those of African-Caribbean descent who return to Barbados usually upon retirement, are labelled by indigenous Barbadians as 'mad English' (Potter and Phillips, 2006: 590). This exclusive imputation is ironically explained as the influence of media coverage of psychiatric diagnosis as it pertains to ethnicity in Britain. In contrast, the differences of other Western 'returnees', specifically those from the USA are normalised by virtue of the perceived cultural (and political) hegemony of North America, over that of Britain (Potter and Phillips, 2006: 596).

At Tranquillity, Chinese susceptibility towards mental illness is frequently seen by Chinese staff as well as by patients as being caused by an excess of mental sophistication as well as frustrated ambition, as exemplified by the person of Jacob in Chapter Four (Chi-Ying Chung *et al.*, 1997). In these accounts the view appears to be that for Chinese migrant communities the struggle to attain material and educational privilege, and the successful outcome of these endeavours in Malaysia, have not acted as a protective factor against mental illness, but indeed in some ways the reverse holds true (Chew, 1999; Ramon, 1996).

In consequence, the outcome of such gross ethnic stereotyping strongly indicates that a significant degree of racism has been commonplace in the hospital setting. One, furthermore, duly noted by patients, such as Maria, a Chinese patient on the private wards, who evidently disliked the Malay nurses who cared for her. She described them as speaking 'harshly' to her and attributed this primarily to the institutionalised under-privileging of Chinese citizens.

> *I don't know why they speak to me like that. Perhaps they think the government belong more to them than to the Chinese. There aren't very many Chinese in power you know. The Dayaks (nurses) are all right but the Chinese nurses are very nice to me, they are motherly and kind.*

Racism at Tranquillity therefore served as a means of moral containment of female and male patients through classification based on cultural values, with Chinese patients being seen to be victimised by their own ethnic group and religious heritage. These patients were viewed by staff as being indisputably social outcasts in a way that Malay and Dayak patients rarely were, and therefore in practical, as well as social and political terms, were consequently easily dismissed as utterly forsaken and therefore inconsequential.

Theories around the issue of 'race'/ethnicity and mental illness have been something of a preoccupation for many psychiatrists working in colonial settings, as has already been noted. Ethnic stereotyping was certainly one of the less savoury aspects of these reflections, in which for instance, Malays were regards as 'over-emotional', North Africans were viewed as likely to become mentally unhinged by their adherence to Islam; and Indonesians, like infants, seemed to have an over-riding need to gratify their desires and with a similar lack of responsibility (Vaughan, 2007:10-11). However, as Vaughan goes on to argue, serious questions were also being raised regarding the universality of mental illness, which later informed the notion of cross-cultural psychiatry (Vaughan, 2007). Along with these issues regarding taxonomies were others, such as the nature and influence of culture on behaviour norms and deviancy; and what would constitute mental illness within given societies, together with what would be seen to alleviate them. In this tradition, we could place much of the published research of Sarawak's alienist Dr Schmidt, in his interest in the protective factors of Dayak community interactions and community interdependence ,in terms of the prognosis of members with mental illness. Nevertheless, as staff accounts here indicate, the teasing out of frankly oppressive attitudes, compared to impartial inquiry into the prevalence of diagnosed mental illness among certain ethnic groups - and predominantly, minority ones - without resorting to racist overtones is a narrow path to tread. A final point worth revisiting lies in the observation that twentieth century psychiatrists in colonial settings were obliged to work within the political context of governance and resistance (Keller, 2001;Vaughan, 2007). Such macro tensions carried repercussions for the mental well being of the subjects of imperialism, as well as in the case of Africa at least, European settlers (McCulloch, 1995; Ernst, 2010). It is debatable how far this observation connects with the continuing socio-political environment enveloping the non-*bumiputera* communities of contemporary Malaysia. Nonetheless, it is one where each individual family are obliged to negotiate the challenges and restrictions that affirmative policies have placed upon their movements and life decisions. Such socio-political circumstances will of necessity demand a high level of competitiveness and tenacity among certain sectors of society for merit to be rewarded fairly; and where not all will show the necessary resilience to achieve and maintain worldly and social success.

Physical containment of the debased

In discussing issues of control and containment on the wards, probably the most tangible evidence of this can be seen in relation to treatment programmes, such as ECT, and through strategies like the use of locked sections on wards. The physical restraining of patients is imposed largely according to the socio-economic status of patients of both sexes, while gender norms, as has been seen, dictate the processes and the means of containment, typified by the conditions under which women patients are kept (Cogliati *et al.*, 1988). From all accounts the rigid demarcations of patient liberty on the grounds of wealth were in place at Hospital Tranquillity since its inception with congested, confined public wards standing in contrast to low numbers on relatively free private wards. These historical distinctions, however, were overturned during one particular period of radical change in the 1980s, in effect a small-scale social revolution, where the walls of the asylum were literally brought down, or at least for many.

The change from the locked to open ward system was the major sweeping reform of Dr Kadir, the previous hospital director, who, inspired by changes taking place in psychiatric institutions in the West, as notably occurred under Basaglia in Italy, sought to create a more liberal environment (Scheper-Hughes and Lovell, 1986). In the hospital, this experimentation with an open ward system has acquired an almost legendary reputation amongst staff, who recall it as being probably the most profound change in the management of patients in their careers.

> Now what has changed is the management, when I was here last time (the undefined past) things were different, patients were very difficult: abusive, assaulting staff. The patients were like animals. I remember one crawling on the ground blind and other people hitting themselves - and they didn't get better. We were afraid of the patients and they were dangerous, unpredictable. But if I were locked up like that I would go mad too.

The reluctance of staff at Tranquillity to embrace these policy changes is reminiscent of similar reactions to the implementation of an open ward system at Fulbourn Hospital in England, where few members of staff were enthusiastic about the changes taking place (Clark, 1996). At Tranquillity, these changes were seen to bring down many of the tangible and perhaps non-tangible barriers that divided patients from their caretakers and were both feared and deplored, as indicated by this account from a medical assistant.

We, the staff were on this side [indicating the small square of the nurses' station] in a cage here. The patients were over there. Our attitudes? Maybe we were afraid. You go in and all the patients are around you. We didn't know the patients. We thought they were the same, all aggressive. But it was much like now in some ways but very depressing ... The floor was concrete and covered in shit, so we had to clean up every day with people just sleeping on the floor.

In interview, Dr Kadir expressed disappointment that in his opinion the open ward system at Hospital Tranquillity was gradually being dismantled over time and fulminates over the current state of affairs.

Can I say that once the ward was opened up there were less incidents of conflict. Now it is becoming closed (again) since (the new director) took over a few years ago. But the staff wasn't happy then. There was a lot of resistance. But I saw that in terms of violence and benefit to the patients, it was better when it was an open ward. Patients could wander around and mingle with the public. And female patients were given open ward access as much as the men.

Most women patients at Tranquillity clearly no longer enjoy this level of freedom in comparison with men on wards. Furthermore, an additional trend noted in the latter months of fieldwork, indicated that male patients in turn were beginning to be subject to confinement in much the same way as women. Whereas previously on Male Ward 1 the grill gate to the hospital corridors was normally left unlocked permitting free access of male patients and visitors on the open ward, more and more frequently I found that the gate was padlocked. When questioned on these changes, medical assistants and particularly junior individuals gave the fear of patients 'absconding' as the primary reason. Thus, it would seem that over the course of time the opportunities of male patients to leave the ward were becoming gradually eroded, as the trend swung back towards a more restrictive model of care. Nevertheless, it is a general truism that fluctuations in these patterns of patient care, would not only be reliant upon contemporary ideologies of care, but particularly heavily dependent upon the attitudes and personalities of hospital directors.

Fear of the oppressed:
Staff accounts of the locked wards

Staff descriptions of conditions on the locked wards of the past are illuminating and harrowing. Long-serving nurses and medical assistants whose careers at Hospital Tranquillity could stem back decades, easily recalled the time when patients were herded behind bars eating, sleeping and defecating on a concrete floor. The conditions under which patients lived were appallingly degrading and inhumane as many members of staff now freely acknowledge. The horrors of working in such a menagerie of the desperate, so similar to historical descriptions of maltreatment, is one that is powerfully recalled by members of staff (Alexander and Selesnick, 1967; Scull, 1979). At Tranquillity under similar circumstances, patients were unable to satisfy even basic instincts for self-care and were therefore seen as closer to beasts than people (Foucault, 1965). Conditions for staff were also poor, albeit to a far lesser extent, where patient faeces, for instance, had to be cleaned up by medical staff without even the benefit of additional cleaning labour or protective gloves. Aggressive incidents towards other patients were common occurrences as were occasional attacks on staff with fear of patients running high.

> We used to be afraid of the patients and they looked at us with a lot of fear. Now it is much better, we are used to working with patients like these... Before the conditions were bad, with patients just lay around on the floor. They had hair lice and skin problems - ringworm very common. Patients were washed with OMO which made their hair stick up like this ...[demonstrates]. Even the diet had been much poorer - it is much better now.

These descriptions conform to traditional concepts of the insane as basically brutish and in need of kennelling tactics and other associated forms of control (Kraepelin, 1962). There was, however, a practical reason behind mass incarceration of patients and this related to the extreme unattractiveness of the nursing task given these appalling conditions.

> There was only one medical assistant and an assistant, sometimes not even an assistant. So how can 1 man see to 40 plus patients? Impossible! So they stayed in the locked ward ... they were very aggressive. Now, there are four medical assistants on the ward, so a patient sees that and doesn't make trouble. If he is aggressive, four of us go in and restrain him. Then, you would be too frightened to go in alone ... the patients are clever they see more staff and they behave better.

The descriptions of early nineteenth century lunatic asylums prior to reform make some telling references to management of the mad due, at least in part, to overcrowding problems. For example, at Bethlem, Scull (1993) states that fifty-two male patients were given over to the care of just a couple of attendants, with an even worse ratio of attendant to patient for females; although evidently this constituted an enviable ratio compared to that described in the above account at Tranquillity. At Bethlem, as well as at other similar lunatic institutions, enforced confinement was used as practically the only means of control, regularly interspersed with episodes of mutual aggression between keeper and inmate, regardless of ineffective attempts by governors to prohibit abuse and maltreatment towards inmates. However, as Scull (1993: 306) adds, the warehousing regime designed to manage large numbers of hapless individuals did not lend itself well to 'initiative and innovation' among the appointed keepers.

Overcrowding and abuse were also correlated in some of the newly built psychiatric resources in Africa (McCulloch, 1995; Jackson, 2005). Sadowsky (1999), for instance, states that based on official reports and witness accounts prior to and following the Second World War conditions in asylums in Nigeria were appalling, where naked, aggressive inmates were chained in congested cells, and effectively treated like wild animals. As already noted in Chapter Six, the problems of patient aggression, congestion and poor facilities, together with a dearth of alternative strategies by staff, appear to have given rise to rigorous types of therapy to control behaviour. Typified by ECT at Tranquillity, this situation is reminiscent of the situation in African asylums were even more extreme forms of control in the form of psychosurgery were practised (McCulloch, 1995).

At Tranquillity, the deplorable state under which patients were kept inevitably created mutual suspicion and fear between staff and patients. Such attitudes can in turn be read as projected fear of the oppressed through the guilt of the oppressor, or those who willingly or reluctantly collude with oppressive systems. The dehumanisation and indeed *demonisation* of psychiatric patients under this kind of regime evidently created severe anxieties amongst staff, compounded by the threat of the removal of the physical barriers that kept these wretched inmates at bay (Clark, 1996).

Circa 2000 the gradual and immediate improvements in care generated by the switch to an open ward have been recognised by staff, but this was often conceded somewhat grudgingly. In reluctant agreement with Dr Kadir, however, long-serving staff commented that the more liberal regime of the open ward did tend to reduce incidents of patient violence. In confirmation, Mary Acton focuses on the comparative rarity of violent attacks by psychiatric patients in the UK, concluding that those most likely to be at risk of such behaviour are normally psychotic with a history of compulsory admissions (Acton, 1990).

A familiar and much publicised concern in the UK has surrounded the question of aggression by psychiatric patients, particularly in relation to community care and the apparent lack of professional supervision. An emphasis on violence on the ward has been proportionately reduced in the public eye, while in the UK a Department of Health report on psychiatric nursing barely mentions the subject (HMSO, 1994). Equally service-user literature has justifiably concentrated on the violence experienced at the hands of staff, rather than the risk of violence to staff (Bell, 1996; Laing, 1996; Rogers *et al.*, 1993). However, just as Elvis on Male Ward 1 expressed a fear of the uncontrollable madman, the staff at Hospital Tranquillity expressed a significant level of anxiety and suspicion of the insane, in which category ironically the timid Elvis, as a patient, would also be included. While violence from women patients was not regarded as a particularly onerous hazard, albeit one that certainly did exist, male patients were singled out as offering the worst level of risk for male and female members of staff (Orme, 1994; Ussher, 1991). In common with social services personnel in the UK, for example, patient abuse of staff at Tranquillity was viewed in terms of actual bodily harm and sexual violence rather than psychological and verbal abuse, which may be regarded as simply part of every-day life (Hester, 1994).

Medical assistants were usually forthcoming with disclosures on the risks of working with the mentally ill, yet it was female nurses who, one might assume, bore the brunt of intimidation by patients on the grounds of gender, and yet at first these very same respondents were the most difficult to engage in discussion. Fortunately these barriers to better understanding of nurses were eventually and unexpectedly overcome and an almost wholehearted embrace replaced the arm's lengthy approach of the nursing sorority towards me. This was a transient but very valuable change in fieldwork relations, culminating in, much to my advantage, some companionable and deeply illuminating discussions on the perceived hazards of the job.

The sequence of events was illuminating in that for the first time on this ward I was invited into the sanctum of the nurses' private coffee room. Here I was allowed to partake in their 'elevenses' while talk flowed freely. The conversation was very revealing and at last I felt invited to be part of their inner group after many months of fieldwork. I complimented myself on my achievement until later upon reflection I realised the true nature behind my apparent breakthrough. Prior to this, I had felt I reached something of an impasse with the nursing staff on this particular ward. My friendly relationships with many of the women patients there tended to militate against being able to form a good working relationship with the staff, who clearly regarded themselves as polarised from patients and were quite suspicious of my motives. Therefore, I felt far from a sense of belonging, so far as my relationship with the nursing staff went, but all this was to change on the morning that I witnessed an assault on a patient. A nurse was in the process of arresting a patient's movement by grabbing her arm through the bars of the locked ward, a struggle then ensued, while the nurse shouted for assistance. Another patient approached her with or without hostile intent and, with her hands, occupied the nurse reacted by pushing her away with what I would describe as a kick to the stomach. I did not see the cause of the scuffle, but I did see the outcome and I was aware that the nurse involved and her colleagues saw me watching. Shortly afterwards I found myself invited to coffee where the topic of the discussion was risk of violence to staff by patients, a subject discussed at length with nurses as being one close to their daily concerns.

My later guess was that the nurses having realised that I had seen an incident that could be fairly described as compromising to the nurse involved, reacted by closing ranks, and in so doing attempted to enclose me as an adopted initiate as well. Over coffee and snacks my understanding was sought in relation to the risks of the job and several examples were given to me of attacks perpetrated on vulnerable members of staff. While my understanding and sympathy was probed, a more valuable commodity at that time may have been my complicity and silence on the incident I had just witnessed.

Nonetheless the insights I developed from this incident and the inclusion I generally experienced on occasions from then on enormously enriched my understanding of what it was like for nurses, and later still for female doctors in the enclosed community of the institution. These accounts differed from those of male staff respondents where to generalise along somewhat stereotypic grounds, men on the whole tended to be reluctant to voice their innermost fears to me, although assailing me with lurid second-hand stories of violent patients. Their experiences remained concealed behind a air of manly fortitude combined with a touch of gallows humour. Typically, experienced medical assistants, especially those on *Bunga Raya ward*, were more likely to exude this type of humour than were junior doctors. Although *Bunga Raya*, the forensic ward, was not generally seen as a popular place to work by staff, its reputation offered compensations. For this ward was seen as being a tough place for tough men and this notoriety rubbed off as a form of exaggerated machismo in the staff, who regarded themselves as 'stronger' than other male personnel in being able to contain their feral charges. In this respect, male madness was viewed stereotypically as far the most threatening in its aggressive manifestations than that demonstrated by women.

> Is it that men's madness is more dangerous, that it somehow needs to be contained, as a wild lion would need to be put behind bars? Is it that because women are expected to be mad, their diagnosis is not a surprise and offers no threat whereas men's does? (Ussher, 1991: 171-2).

Additionally, in keeping with its forensic feature, Bunga Raya was also seen as 'more important than other wards - because the medical report is based on our observations', as one member of staff put it. In other words, the professional observations of the medical assistants could help to make the difference between incarceration in a prison or a hospital - or indeed between life and a State-mandated death sentence. Accordingly, this kind of professional responsibility generated interest in the inmates; and certainly did no harm to the self-esteem and general reputation of their keepers. On the whole, staff on *Bunga Raya* therefore demonstrated fewer effects of demoralisation in comparison with staff on other wards. Equally, however, they showed a reluctance to reveal any perceived weakness of character in the interview situation, with a consequent lack of detailed information on violence towards staff on the forensic ward.

Cunning and deceit: The essentialised patient

Doctors, especially junior doctors, working in the outpatient clinic were more likely to emphasise the potential dangers of dealing with psychotic patients than the nursing staff. One drew my attention to the lack of an alarm in the clinic and the awkward and potentially dangerous access arrangements of consulting cubicles. Clearly this individual was unhappy about the hospital's policies towards ensuring staff safety, following a recent assault on another doctor. Because doctors primarily deal with a large number of psychotic patients who require assessment before admission to the ward, the risk of violence from this group is higher than from patients in the public-ward situation. By contrast, however, nursing staff of both sexes were more likely to express the greatest anxiety over non-psychotic psychiatric patients. These differences reflect the roles of medical staff, whereby nursing staff daily deal with a variety of patients, of whom the psychotic patients normally form a minority. Nursing staff were much more preoccupied with issues of daily supervision and the risks associated with that role.

Nursing accounts from both male and female nurses were remarkably similar in describing the assumed essential nature of psychiatric patients. This was often depicted in stereotypic and dualist terms, of being irrational yet calculating, devoid of commonsense yet devious. In this regard, such discourses were not dissimilar to those that prevailed in the eighteenth century, where despite the rationalism of the age and the rise of 'moral treatment' the mad were still viewed as fundamentally ferocious but cowardly (Scull, 1993). Accordingly, at Tranquillity ward staff frequently conveyed the risk involved in taking patients to task over misdemeanours as offering an opportunity for retaliation on unsuspecting staff. It was made clear to me that it was important therefore for staff not to be lulled into a false sense of security or to place themselves at a disadvantage in terms of maintaining discipline, as this account from a nurse on the acute female ward indicates.

> *If the patients see you understaffed then they try to challenge you ....Yes, they remember when you have to restrain them, but they may not remember the details but they remember who they don't like.*

Similar accounts from nursing staff on the male and female wards all focused on the treachery of patients, who, when the time seemed opportune might suddenly attack for injuries real or imagined. This was exemplified through the experiences of Sister Weng who was punched in the stomach by a male patient in a fit of rage 'because his wife had left him'; and Sister Angela who was hit in the mouth with a cup of water she had handed to a patient.

Patients, I was given to understand, are 'clever', they approach 'behind your back' when staff are alone or with their attention on other tasks. This kind of discourse concentrated on the deceit and treachery of the subordinated, and reflected the uneasiness staff felt over the prevailing discrepancies of power. The *status quo* ensures that patients feel regularly helpless: a patient can be surrounded and overpowered by several members of staff, then subjected to various indignities and physical trials, without recourse to negotiation or effective protest. The portrayal of psychiatric patients as essentially amoral, opportunist, fundamentally dangerous and anti-social justified, therefore, the measures of control regularly meted out by staff. These perceptions therefore lent themselves to a tendency towards the custodial, as noted by the nursing body SNMAC (1999) in the UK. The swings in ward policy towards the conservative and disciplinary, unequally balanced by moves towards more liberal regimes, did little to allay staff fear of patients, resulting in 'crack-downs' and a continuous and vicious circle of the associated dread of the oppressed.

Violence towards female staff

It would be unfair, however, to dismiss staff fears as exaggerated or misplaced given the evident seriousness of some of the attacks, particularly those inflicted on female staff by male patients (Hester, 1994). Personal experiences of violence were offered by female staff respondents among doctors and nurses; for example this account from one of the most experienced and approachable of the long-serving nurses:

> *Last time I was attacked was in 1996, I was directing a patient to the admission room but he looked lost so I said, 'never mind, I'll take you there'. On the way he suddenly hit me violently in the head and I was knocked unconscious, and then he beat me in the belly and in the head with his fists. I heard about all this from the people in OT (occupational therapy ward) who saw my legs kicking around, even though I was still unconscious. I was given 2 days sick leave by the doctor and told to go home. I had headaches for a year and a half and I think it all had a bad effect on my memory, it's not so good anymore.*

The violence perpetrated on women members of staff can be viewed as an occupational hazard in dealing with male psychiatric patients who victimise the women professionals, who embody a wider system of control whilst being personally vulnerable to attack (Hester, 1994). Abuse is furthermore compounded through institutional responses and collegial attitudes as this account from a still traumatised female doctor indicates.

> *I had a very bad experience in January when I was beaten up, perhaps you heard? He (the patient) was just sitting across from me like this. Usually everything is OK, you get a bit anxious once in a while, but he just went! He grabbed my hair and pounded my head into the glass on my desk. I screamed, luckily, and one of the MAs came in and pulled him off me. It was pretty nasty; actually I mean no bones broken but the trauma, the fear. (The director) came down and said 'take a few days off', but I had enough people saying by Monday, this happened on a Wednesday, [imitates sighing impatience] 'You fall off a horse you get back on', and*

I'm saying, 'I don't need this!' But when I take time off, it's just a loan, so I came back to work too soon. X (male colleague) has apologised for this, his social skills aren't so good anyway, but his idea of supporting me is he sat beside me, the day I returned and critiques how I am dealing with patients at that time. I mean talk of interpersonal skills! I am traumatised! Shut down! My interpersonal skills were not the best that day, I mean after that I leave the hospital in tears.

Findings based on staff accounts indicated that at Tranquillity little awareness of staff anxieties was demonstrated at a managerial level. Consequently issues like rapid response and standard alarm systems seemed to be at a rudimentary level of implementation and poorly applied. If male doctors and medical assistants found the current system inadequate, women members of staff were evidently even more at risk of attack, and in addition to the risk of beatings were also subject to sexual violence by male patients.

I was going to the toilet, but not the staff toilet but the one for the public because it was nearer. There was a man from the out-patients (clinic), a patient, and I didn't see him but he came in after me, pushed in after I got into the toilet and knocked me onto the floor, he tore my baju (shirt/jacket). Well, of course, I kicked him but he was on top of me. I saw his 'thing' ready to enter ...it was horrible! I didn't tell anyone for three days, I was too afraid he would find out and come back.

Based on these narratives my detection and increasing awareness of a sense of pervading vulnerability in staff began to erode my own trust of patient participants to some degree. Previously in undertaking fieldwork, I experienced many different emotions but none of these could be described as fear, as such. A sense of my own personal safety had been formed through a naïve belief that I was obviously a well-meaning individual, whilst relying heavily on my outsider status as being removed from the 'vectors of power' played out in the hospital system (Narayan, 1997: 31).

Following interviews with staff on occupational risk at Tranquillity I found that I began to feel vulnerable in the presence of some patients, not all men by any means, and in parts of the hospital where previously I had felt perfectly safe, although not necessarily always comfortable. The caution that nurses now began to urge on me in my interactions with patients altered my perception of inviolability, and went some way to creating distance between patient participants and myself. The somewhat disconcerting habit, for instance, of seemingly harmless, grandmotherly Luwee in her tendency to approach me from behind and catch me in an enveloping embrace now began to assume more sinister overtones. It was only later that I learned that Luwee had been obliged to relocate to Tranquillity after scalding her elderly neighbour to death by pouring a boiling kettle over him. On another occasion, I was quite shaken to find a patient standing directly behind me during an interview when a nurse began suddenly to indicate this by warning gestures. To my shame, I discovered it was none other than Soo Mei from Female Ward 1 who wanted to bid me an emotional, final farewell as she was about to be discharged and realised she would not be seeing me again. A similar, and thankfully as it turned out, uneventful incident, took place with a male patient on *Bunga Raya* ward, which had by now become an almost welcoming and friendly place to me, despite its sobering, reputation for holding serious offenders. On this occasion, an intense and intelligent acquaintance had, unknown to me, followed me into an empty, secluded room I had wandered into. I turned to find him staring contemplatively at me and for a brief, but pulse-pausing moment, he seemed intent on preventing me leaving, until suddenly he dropped the bar of his arm and allowed me to leave unharmed and very relieved.

Although I experienced no personal attacks, the watchful nervousness that I began to develop at one point, almost entirely through being influenced by staff accounts of violence, was illuminating. The anxiety that staff conveyed prevented them forming friendly and trusting relationships with patients, while instead the theme of the duplicity and veiled hostility of patients ran as a common warning amongst them, and was duly imparted to new members of staff (Higgins *et al*, 1999). The official response to violence towards staff in its inadequate and indeed almost callous indifference permitted staff anxieties to grow and fester. This in turn led to hardening of attitudes in staff towards their own vulnerabilities and those of colleagues, with resulting repercussions on their emotional resilience towards managing patients and the job in general. Women professionals at Tranquillity were seen to be particularly vulnerable to the institutionalised response to abuse, as summed up by a weary although angry response from this woman doctor.

Being a woman here? It has its plus and has its minuses. It has its pluses because the male staff (MAs) look out for me. Dr Jerry said, 'You've got to take charge!' But he's a man, I mean I'm sorry but its fine for a 6ft something guy, I mean I didn't bother to tell him that, but if you can't see that there's a difference because I am a woman and smaller. I mean sometimes the patients go for me, and the MAs say 'Dr P go away!' It has its pluses as I say, but it has its minuses, they (MAs) may not take me as seriously as male colleagues. So being a woman, protects me – it makes me less effective, but it protects me.

Female doctors at Tranquillity attempted to claim a rightful position of authority that was nonetheless seen to be an anomaly on the grounds of gender, the majority of women occupying a significantly lower position in the medical hierarchy. Consequently, while being expected to demonstrate the behaviour and standards of control over staff and patients that senior male colleagues demanded, they were awarded less professional credibility *as* women. The result of this was that medical assistants might react protectively towards women doctors at a personal level, while hospital policies and systems did not appear to offer particularly effective protection towards either female or male members of staff. Instead a hard-boiled collegial attitude of 'if you can't stand the heat get out of the kitchen' was imposed by senior, male doctors on junior doctors of both sexes and this impacted heavily on the morale of these members of staff.

Although anxiety and trauma appeared to be better handled by women nurses in the exclusively female company of other nurses, nonetheless the masculinised values prevalent in the hospital hierarchy prevented these from being validated in the wider context of work. Feelings of vulnerability therefore seemed to remain unendorsed and poorly supported with resulting symptoms of 'burn-out' evident in many members of staff, and conveyed in interviews, particularly with women and male junior doctors (Higgins *et al.*, 1999: 76-7). The level of open disillusion with the work varied amongst staff, but appeared to be rife amongst junior doctors of both sexes, whose notions regarding the care and treatment of people with mental illnesses had undergone the greatest change in expectation since beginning work at Tranquillity. Nurses and medical assistants did not voice this level of disillusion, but conveyed that their more pessimistic views had been borne out by their experiences and that consequently less of a professional and attitudinal adjustment had been made towards their charges over time. A uniting factor amongst doctors and nursing staff was a notably cynical and weary attitude towards the remedial care of recalcitrant psychiatric patients. For the majority of staff the perception was that little could be offered but accommodation and containment, with an associated emphasis on the need for staff to cover their backs and retain control at all times.

The cloistered containment of patients in many psychiatric hospitals, like Tranquillity, create a claustrophobic environment that entraps members of staff who are thereby designated the role of keeper rather than therapist. Accordingly, in keeping with the rationale and rhythms of the asylum care imposed, the preoccupation of staff is to keep the system running as smoothly as possible, partially by ensuring that security is constantly observed. Routine medical or nursing tasks must therefore be viewed as potential areas of risk; and staff are aware from personal or secondary experience that attempts to personalise care may backfire dangerously. New staff are quickly acculturated into this focus on risk and the need to be wary of their charges on the ward, to the extent where they may feel they cannot afford to let their guard down at all.

Systems so entrenched in long established regimentation, such as the asylum, do not easily adapt to change, and progressive staff like Zulhan, the MA, can find themselves swimming against the tide in their attempt to humanise relationships with patients and to provide rehabilitative exercises. This is no easy option given the rigid hierarchy of medical roles among doctors, nurses and MAs, that are themselves embedded within a comparably ossified system as that of the asylum.

9
Towards community psychiatry

Like all psychiatric hospitals in the country, Hospital Tranquillity is currently positioned somewhat uncomfortably at a cusp of change in mental health provision that is slowly taking place in Malaysia. Although it is some years since reform of current mental health legislation was first put forward, these have yet to complete their gradual progress through the Parliament and be fully enacted. Thus, it appears that little has changed on the landscape of mental health policy and psychiatric practice in the last decade. The planned revisions, however, remain generally intact and just as psychiatric care has roots in the country's colonial past; a course that runs parallel with Western developments continues to steer the general direction of contemporary services. Therefore, the current if theoretical trajectory for mental-health services in Malaysia is moving towards the decentralisation of psychiatric hospitals, albeit at a haphazard pace (Ashencaen Crabtree and Chong, 2001).

In the European context, the move towards community-based care forms an uneven continuum encouraging the greater democratisation of psychiatry, articulated as a civil-rights and humanitarian move (Campbell, 1996). The closure of institutional care in keeping with the ideology behind care in the community, has nevertheless been contested. One argument posits that those individuals with long term mental health needs may actually require the refuge (or asylum) of long term institutional care. This point is expanded by Deva (2004: 172) who notes that patients are seen as best served within psychiatric institutions, as opposed to psychiatric wings in general hospitals, as short-term care is likely to be less 'meaningful', owing to the concentration of psychiatric expertise in long stay psychiatric institutions, like Tranquillity. Furthermore, insufficient resources have been made available by Western governments to enable community-based care to be effectively enacted (Payne, 1995). Human rights discourses, however, have to-date over-ridden these objections, although the community care experiment has yet to reach its ultimate conclusion.

At Tranquillity, by contrast, as an example of institutional care in Malaysia, paradigms from seemingly quite incompatible eras of Western psychiatric care were imposed simultaneously and imploded into a confusion

---

of rhetorical stances that appeared to keep progress immobilised and the condition of patients static. This is a situation noted by Rostom and Lee (1996) in their study of major psychiatric service providers on the Peninsula.

> We were informed that the recent policy in decentralisation only extends to the concept of relocating services outside the hospital for care in the community projects, it does not appear to encompass the wider issues of service-user empowerment (Rostom and Lee, 1996: 25).

The low-key rationale for decentralisation in Malaysia has, as has the UK, been subject to budgetary concerns, where it was hoped that this would be a cost-effective approach to care (Ashencaen Crabtree and Chong, 2001). However, it might be more to the point to see decentralisation in Malaysia as an attempt to keep abreast of contemporary developments in psychiatric-service provision, but subject to ideological qualifications removed from emancipatory goals (Campbell, 1996; Scheper-Hughes and Lovell, 1986). Furthermore, as Forrester-Jones points out in her study of community care moves in Britain, the unpalatable fact is that doubtless there will always be some individuals who will require semi-permanent residential care. As the largest majority of patients at Hospital Tranquillity are so perceived, little, in consequence is felt necessary in the way of fundamental changes to the current system (Forrester-Jones, 1995: ii). As Sue Estroff points out, de-institutionalisation in itself does not remove the fundamental barriers of social exclusion faced by psychiatric patients.

> De-institutionalisation has, for the most part, been simplistically effected through movement away from the architectural embrace of hospitals. But institutions, of course, are complex, extending beyond walls to the articulation of traditions and values at a societal level. In this sense, the institutions of chronic mental illness have been little affected by the escape from institutional buildings. The roles, expectations, stereotypes, and responses that accompany being a back-ward patient or a long-term community outpatient have changed little (Estroff, 1981: 253-254).

While the upper hierarchy promote community psychiatry as the prevalent future model of care, this is by no means a unanimous view. At Tranquillity many members of staff were sceptical of the projected vision of community psychiatry, whilst others appeared quite oblivious to the concepts that formed a bone of contention 'upstairs'.

In interview in 2000, the hospital director spoke enthusiastically about

Tranquillity's future, describing an exciting community-based service that would take place under the 8th Malaysia Plan scheduled for the coming five years (Malaysia, 1991; Malaysia, 1993). Ambitious projected plans included the building of a new two-storey fifty-six-bed, acute block at the general hospital, a day hospital and community psychiatric nursing facilities. The grounds of Tranquillity itself would house the siting of a new polyclinic covering outpatient appointments, thus allowing downsizing of the hospital to accommodate chronic and other long-stay patients only, a practical plan in view of the predominantly chronic patient population. Unfortunately, some snags were encountered early this century which hindered these exciting developments, the first being the need to obtain permission to proceed from the Sarawak State Government: a major problem in itself. Any concern on this front was well-founded as subsequently the Sarawak State Government rejected the plans outright without giving formal reasons, although the low priority given to psychiatric patients and, by association, their professional attendants, was generally regarded as being at the root of the matter.

Before this blow fell, however, it seemed at the time that the other major issue revolved around taking the first steps into the unknown unaided by government advice, much to the director's despair.

Nobody seems to know how to go about it, lah. It means more than just decentralising the hospitals ... (it) means providing services in the community: day care, day hospitals, community services like halfway home. Unfortunately promoting mental-health issues rather than community psychiatry as such ... although promoting is part of community psychiatry, but it doesn't provide services for those who are mentally distressed!

While plans for decentralised services in Sarawak are nominally driven by hospital directors under a political mandate, the implementation of such a large-scale project lies primarily through a coalition with the 'coal-face' nursing staff. Ironically, it was these very individuals who seemed the least informed about or involved in plans afoot. This situation was not aided by the fact that there was a conspicuous lack of specific and accountable guidelines published and disseminated by government agencies on the matter (Ashencaen Crabtree and Chong, 2001). Consequently, the plans to integrate acute psychiatric-service provision with general hospital services required a certain evangelism on the part of its advocates.

The delegation of the necessary roles required for success in implementing community services was by no means a simple matter and involved negotiating a whole panorama of turf boundaries. One prominent psychiatrist and active proponent of the decentralisation move in Malaysia, expressed impatience with the attitude of the front-line personnel designated for the task of bringing about community services. This group was described as being already engaged in dealing indirectly with community mental-health needs, but nonetheless shying away from casting these activities into a formal and directly interventionist role.

> *They won't handle the mental-health cases but will refer out. In terms of mental health, they are doing it (psychiatric work), but the personnel don't recognise it. When this programme came in (decentralisation), there is a lot of dissatisfaction: fear of extra work. If the mental-health programme is being established - implemented properly - they are scared that they won't have time, training. But they don't need extra time, it is no extra work to them, they have these cases anyway. They believe that it is extra work: 'My work is this!' They want this (mental health) to be specialised, to be handled by special doctors, but there are many other diseases which are not handled by specialised people.*

The recalcitrant professionals that this individual spoke of with irritation were the public-health medical assistants employed in a variety of care sectors including, for instance, the male wards at Hospital Tranquillity. This, however, only reflected some of the problems for the implementation of community-based care, which required a concerted, co-ordinated approach from the health authorities and social services, as noted by this affiliated NGO worker:

> *The Welfare Department regards mental illness as a medical problem, there's no perception of psychosocial needs at a practical social-work level. There's a very poor alliance between health and welfare. In theory they should be involved but ... There is a community mental health policy but nothing concrete. Critical services, accommodation support, sheltered employment crisis intervention teams – none of that being done through the Government sector; NGOs are providing in that area on a very small scale, you know.*

Problems ran deeper however, where abrogation of responsibility by the social services has hardly been open to effective challenge. In the meantime, a more fundamental structural problem has existed in which, while all psychiatrists belong to the health sector, community mental health comes under the public health sector, leaving it unclear which Government departments are responsible for implementing community care.

Turf boundaries then acted as a general obstacle in the way of providing satisfactory community support, which Government plans and proclamations appeared to do little to tackle (Ashencaen Crabtree and Chong, 1999b). The general response of the social services has been a refusal to acknowledge any real role in the care of psychiatric patients in the community, while NGOs continue to take up the slack in service provision. In this somewhat chaotic situation, it is hardly surprising that hospital personnel were regarded, and, as will be seen, portrayed themselves as unmotivated to do other than keep Tranquillity ticking over much in the way it has done for years.

Dissent in the ranks

The major problem for community-based service lay in the simple fact that it requires members of staff other than the architects of these plans to carry out the services. At Tranquillity, the hospital plans consequently hinged on the nursing teams in their various capacities to realise these ambitious plans, while these roles were moreover based in part upon professionally restrictive gender normative roles.

A dominant branch of the nursing resource that is essential to community-based care is the hospital's CPNs (Community Psychiatric Nurses), and where notably, their workload doubled in volume during the period of my fieldwork. Accordingly, CPN intervention is considered essential to managing outpatient care in Malaysia (Lau and Hardin, 1996). The CPN team at Tranquillity consisted of two nurses and a medical assistant who were reliant on a driver, and at that time, a rather dilapidated vehicle to make regular forays into the decidedly beautiful but inaccessible rural outback. Unfortunately, due to budgeting constraints it was not seen as possible to increase the number of staff from its original team size of three people, as this would also require additional transport that the hospital could not afford. These kinds of practical issues were trivial but substantially significant blocks to progress, which created their own frustrations as articulated to me by the outraged barks from a visiting nursing practitioner who demanded to know 'But where is the vision? Where is the planning?' A question that of necessity had to remain at least temporarily unanswered.

Accordingly, the pressures of the job consequently grew and while members of the team audibly approved of the pivotal role they would be playing, in interview one of the nurses pointed out some of the difficulties ahead, particularly in relation to the benefit of medical assistants over that of nurses in the nature of their official capacity.

CPN: Only Michael (CPN) can prescribe medication, *as* a medical assistant. We can't because we are nurses, we cannot even prescribe Panadol! If Michael is on leave then we must find a doctor able to prescribe ... and this takes so much time with so many patients and appointments.

Researcher: Would you say this was an example of sexism in the services; the way nurses and medical assistants have different duties like this?

CPN: Maybe. But the system has always been like that.

In Malaysia, the male-dominated medical profession retains a very high status and an authority that is largely unchallenged by the public or allied professions. Psychiatry accordingly carries these gender biases as well the privileges of medical status, although arguably to a lesser extent due to the perceived stigma of mental health (Selig, 1988). Consequently, the power of the profession in Malaysia remains unquestioned by allied professions, such as psychology, occupational therapy and social work; and is comparable to the situation affecting psychiatric staff, other than actual psychiatrists, in the British context (Ramon, 1988: 10).

Although nurses and medical assistants undertake similar duties on the ward, their motives for this line of work are characteristically somewhat different. In the general health setting in Malaysia nurses and medical assistants occupy specifically designated gendered roles, whereby 'nurses' are always women, and are largely assigned a skilled but supportive and subordinate role to those of male colleagues. However, the medical training of medical assistants being men reflects the dominant view that as it is men who largely occupy the elite profession of medicine this rubs off on medical assistants. They in turn can expect a different level of training that conforms to a superior stereotype. This stands in some contrast to the situation in Britain whereby

> The right to make a diagnosis and prescribe a form of treatments is a core element of the professional power of doctors, jealously guarded from encroachment by other clinical staff such as nurses (Barnes and Bowl, 2001: 60).

The incorporation of medical knowledge with a view to prescribing medications demonstrates that medical assistants are inherently expected to carry more responsibility than nurses do, and are more closely affiliated with the kudos that is attached to doctors. It is medical assistants therefore who run the rural polyclinics prevalent in Sarawak. This is considered a challenging and responsible post, where initiative and independence are demanded at a high level. Accordingly, at Hospital Tranquillity selected medical assistants and doctors work alongside each other in the outpatient clinic examining, prescribing and admitting patients, with the doctors assessing new and/or complicated cases. Nurses, including female CPNs, were therefore not considered professionally competent to undertake the responsibility of prescribing even basic medication by virtue of their different training and roles (Witz, 1992).

Community psychiatry and coal-face staff

The special role carved out for medical assistants in the Malaysian health care system emphasises their vital role in creating viable community psychiatric services. The implications behind these expectations, however, seemed to have made little impact on these same individuals at Hospital Tranquillity and stood quite at odds with their plans and perception of their role in psychiatric nursing. A logical guess would further suggest that if the conditions of work differ for nurses and medical assistants it is likely that the rewards and reasons for choosing work in a psychiatric institution also differed for men and women respectively. In both groups, however, the majority of nursing staff of either sex were only recently appointed due to a number of long-serving nurses and medical assistants now reaching retirement age.

For the new arrivals, a point in common lay in the fact that usually they had not specifically entertained ambitions to work in psychiatric nursing. Most of these individuals had been transferred to the hospital from other parts of Malaysia, and not necessarily with their full consent, while others had chosen to come for a variety of reasons both personal and professional.

Hospital Tranquillity is a resource that is continuously short-staffed to a greater or lesser extent; and in Malaysia medical staff can be transferred to wherever they are needed with little regard to people's preferences, hence staffing levels fluctuated around a core of established members, depending on the migration and departure of staff. Fortunately, as the hospital is located in a desirable city with good living standards, reluctant staff usually find that they are compensated in terms of quality of life for working in an environment which otherwise may not have been their first choice.

Rather than remain deployed in the kind of rural backwaters that would soon be targeted for community services several of the medical assistants had opted to transfer to centralised health vacancies in the city and had consequently found themselves placed at Hospital Tranquillity. That the running of these rural clinics was evidently a tough and undesirable occupation is made clear in the following account from a medical assistant.

> *This is like a holiday after the clinics. I am talking about the small rural clinics not the big polyclinics. I used to do everything - the cleaning, the grass cutting, the diagnosis, treatment and then being on call at night. Very tough work, you can work all night and then all the next day. At Tranquillity, we do the same work as the nurses and just follow the doctor's orders – more relaxing.*

Rural clinics are the backbone of primary health care in Sarawak, where rugged terrain separates small, isolated communities (Ashencaen Crabtree and Chong, 1999c). Medical assistants assigned to these clinics are responsible for their day-to-day running and are therefore likely to see a wide variety of cases, referring on to general and specialist resources when patient conditions exceed their professional competence. This, however, was regarded as an onerous task and one not likely to improve with the advent of community services. At least in the hospital, ran the implication, psychiatry followed a predictable and well-worn path that was unlikely to overwhelm the expertise and energies of staff, as indicated in this account:

Field notes. Male Ward 1

'I like it (the job) – much easier than in the clinic before …Then there was only me and one other fellow to do everything, *lah*! People would come any time – night, day, it was very busy. Here we just look after the patients and follow doctors' orders and you can talk with patients! …. But sometimes you cannot. I just follow orders here and the patients obey us when we tell them to do things, *lah*. No, I did not choose to come here, I wanted to go to XGH (general hospital) but - I will stay for a little while, maybe I will go for training like Zulhan (another MA). It is good here and close to X, where I live, so ….'

Zulhan was an outstanding example of a competent, trained and more importantly enthusiastic individual, and much appreciated by patients like Jacob. Zulhan's type of psychiatric nursing was therefore seen by some patients to be a dynamic and skilled role model for other members of staff, and one that went a long way in improving the lot of the patient population (Barnes and Bowl, 2001). Zulhan's methods, however, were not seen as a norm of nursing standards for Tranquillity that medical assistants unanimously cared to aspire to. Instead, a rather less energetic role was the one on which most medical assistants chose to model their intervention. Most medical assistants who had transferred to the hospital from the difficult working environments of clinics seemed to a man to be delighted to find themselves in the relatively unpressurised, and indeed in some respects, even 'cushy' berth, after the humdrum, exhausting life of the rural clinics.

The development of community services was not a topic therefore that was raised by these respondents as relevant to their understanding and practice of nursing care in a psychiatric hospital. Many medical assistants at Tranquillity had opted to step down from a professional role that was demanding but autonomous, and copy a more traditional nursing model that was premised on a conventional subordination to medical officers. Far from expressing resentment about being relegated to a role of *just* 'following' medical orders, many medical assistants actually found their supervisory role a very welcome relief from the burdensome chore of treatment in the wider community, rather than a form of professional emasculation.

Therefore, and unsurprisingly, their views of psychiatric nursing were unprogressive in many ways. Ward life for male patients, unlike the experiences of these medical assistants, could not be regarded as a reprieve, and particularly for those on the chronic wards, this tended towards the regimented. Medical assistants often openly adopted a supervisory role that seemed based on the mundane existence of the military barracks in peace-time:

Field notes. Male Ward 2

The ward is very 'spick-and-span', all beds are made up in the same fashion. The MA explains that the patients and staff make the beds and a lot of attention is given to them being made just *so*, sheets spread tight, single white blanket folded at the end, pillows facing in the same direction. The opening to the pillowcase is meant to face left, although apparently and provokingly not all of them do. He asks me what I think of the ward, I think he expects some praise; I find it hard to find the right words. Finally I say it is very tidy, and comment that the beds are made up as you might find in an army barracks - maybe not the best thing to say, as he looks at me askance.

The imposition on patients of pointless but exact exercises, such as precision bed-making, reinforces their loss of self-determination, as noted by Goffman (1991). Additionally for the outsider, the *ceremonialisation* of the enclosed universe that is institutional life, confirms the belief that theirs is an enclosed universe premised on concepts and governed by rules that are utterly removed from, and alien to, a more normalised existence (Goffman, 1991). The 'military model' imposed at Tranquillity once again draws parallels with Britain in the early twentieth century where similar conditions could be found in Severalls Hospital, as this extract indicates.

> The chief male nurse ... played more of the role of a military commander than one having any *familial* associations (my italics). Discipline was firm and the regimes strict ... (Gittins, 1998: 99).

Despite the somewhat bizarre nature of regimented routines imposed by medical assistants as a main duty in their nursing role, the tempo at the hospital from the staff point of view, was regarded as soothing *and* containable. Better still, it appeared to stand in sharp contrast to the conditions of the rural clinics; and was, as one informant says, an easy-going life in which there was little to do and consequently little expected of patients.

In common once more with Severall's Hospital of a much earlier era, few nurses found work at Tranquillity as attractive as some of their male counterparts did (Gittins, 1998). Most of the younger generation of nurses felt that their preferred position was back in general nursing practice, but that often events had conspired to ensure that they served a term at this hospital. Unlike many of their older and more experienced counterparts there was little commitment shown to psychiatric nursing; and consequently little enthusiasm was expressed for the practical considerations of community-based care, as noted by this dubious respondent:

> *Relatives put patients into hospital (general hospital). They want them to be safe. I don't think they will like our patients being there. It will be a problem ... maybe chronic patients would be better.*

It was considered understandable amongst nurses that the general public would not wish to rub shoulders with psychiatric patients in general hospital settings. Two particular reasons were offered for this view, one being the notoriety of psychiatric patients as incorrigibly unpredictable and violent, and the second being the time worn stigma associated with mental illness.

If community-based care was not generally regarded by nurses as offering an invigorating and liberating alternative to the current scenario of institutional care, the hospital itself was also regarded as an equally unattractive prospect for nurses. Some participants declared that the best place to be, professionally speaking, was on the sick ward where nurses were able to carry out basic nursing tasks very similar to those that they had been trained for in general hospital practice and with no consequent loss of skills in those areas. In interview nurses frequently expressed the fear of becoming deskilled in comparison with general nursing colleagues elsewhere. Furthermore, in agreement with the views of medical assistants, the perception from nurses was that there was little else to do but 'supervise the patients' and 'give out medications': patients generally requiring some form of additional professional expertise that could not be met through basic nursing practice.

In addition, most young nurses did not appear to find the different professional expectations attached to their role a particularly doubtful practice. The issue of the greater medical responsibility given to medial assistants, at least in terms of prescribing medication as opposed to following medical orders, was apparently accepted as unproblematic. Nurse perceptions of these gender differences in the professions appeared to conform to the comfortable notion of *equal* but *different*; and the 10% extra 'critical allowance' that they received in their pay packets as a token of their essential status in hospitals acknowledged this difference. In turn, these views tended to uphold Karim's assertion that gender roles in Malaysia are 'bilateral' and complementary and do not conform to analyses of gender bias because they are not subject to defined positions of hierarchy, as in the West (Karim, 1995: 36). Yet, at the same time, the account given by the CPN points towards the reduced effectiveness of nurses based on these differences; thus indicating a factual, if not perceived, repercussion of institutional sexism in the medical hierarchy that has long been a feature in the health professions historically.

At Tranquillity, with the presumption that time hung heavily on their hands, nurses on the acute and chronic wards were seen working alongside female patients for hours on end, engrossed in the most monotonous of the 'female' occupational therapy tasks, such as the 'thread-sorting' chores. Perhaps overtly this was to provide an industrious example to patients; I, however, viewed it as providing an interesting example of how the barriers between nurses and female patients could be blurred to a minor but significant degree. In comparison, however bored they might confess to being, medical assistants usually observed the distinctions of rank, maintained their distance with patients, and did not seem to participate in the occupational therapy work and general chores regularly allotted to patients.

Despite the discontent of many nurses, several stated that they had managed to find sufficient compensation in the job to outweigh its shortcomings, at least in the short term. Becoming deskilled, however, could be seen to be a very real danger for nurses and one that was duly recognised by visiting nursing students from the local university.

I think things are different from what I expected. Well, we came here to see if the theory we learn in college is like it is at the hospital ... and it's different I think. It doesn't fit. There's not much happening on the ward. Maybe it's the management's fault. There's OT, but if you're not stable? No, I don't want to go into psychiatric nursing when I graduate, I want to work in a (general) hospital and get lots of experience.

The students' general disenchantment with the reality of nursing at the hospital, compared to expectations derived from classroom tuition, was compounded through the advantage of comparisons with other hospitals on the Peninsula, as one student stated:

This place is much more like a mental hospital, like an asylum. There's no stimulation for patients here, maybe they should have things like behaviour therapy, relaxation therapy and group therapy.

Evidently therefore, nurses and medical assistants at Tranquillity tended to jointly regard the job of psychiatric nursing as being fundamentally concerned with supervision rather than with therapeutic tasks. Because of this ambitious staff amongst the nurses were unlikely to consider psychiatric nursing as anything other than a temporary departure from mainstream and more socially valued work in the health services.

Just as medical assistants resigned themselves to working at the hospital for personal and practical reasons, some of the younger nurses offered explanations of domestic convenience as a reason for temporarily accepting a post at the hospital. To reiterate, close to the hospital lies an army barracks and it was quite commonplace, if somewhat incongruous, to find army personnel eating in the *al fresco* hospital canteen. The association between the army barracks and the hospital was maintained not so much through the quality of the hospital dining facilities one guesses, but more likely due to the fact that several of the younger nurses were married to army officers. These nurses, however, were birds of passage, moving from one post to another across a wide variety of health resources according to their husband's army transfers and consequently stayed for a brief season only. Nurses like these were prepared to transfer to other postings across the country as required by the army and their husbands, for as one nurse put it: 'wives follow husbands, not husbands wives'.

There were mixed opinions on how this affected nurses' attitudes to work and careers: few had an abiding interest in psychiatric nursing as such, while psychiatric training amongst nursing staff was a rarity. Less than a bare handful of nurses and medical assistants had completed specialist mental health training; a deficiency that was only partially met by attempts at in-house training and plans to access long-distance courses from the West and the Asia Pacific region. Consequently, some nurses maintained that it was better to keep moving and get general experience beyond psychiatry. Others admitted that constant transfers tended to jeopardise their attempts to climb the promotional ladder, although this served their husbands' careers well.

At Tranquillity, however, many nurses felt unable to fully utilise their basic nursing skills; and seemed in general not to have acquired a compensatory new set specific to their role in psychiatric care. That this was true of the medical assistants as well offered no consolation, and postings such as this one to Tranquillity appeared to do little more for most than swell their *curriculum vitae* to some extent, in readiness for better opportunities elsewhere.

Making a difference?
Social work and counselling

For some years Hospital Tranquillity had benefited from social work services, originally provided through VSO (Voluntary Services Overseas) support, but more recently in the form of a small social work team in addition to a hospital counsellor, all consisting of young women who were still in the experimental stage of consolidating career options. In Malaysia, counselling has carved a more prominent foothold in the professions than social work has yet managed to do (Baba *et al.*, 2010). Counsellors therefore are more likely to have some higher recognised professional standing and training than social workers. Yet, or perhaps because of these circumstances, in interview the counsellor then employed conveyed that she primarily focused on the families of patients, rather than patients themselves, as these were not seen as being able to benefit particularly from counselling therapy on the grounds of their disorders and lack of insight. Families by contrast were regarded as requiring a lot of emotional support to continue their onerous involvement with relatives with mental illnesses whose needs were by comparison seen as of lesser priority. Views from Male Ward 1 regarding the counselling service differed markedly, with Teo, for instance, grumbling that neither he nor anyone else on the ward had ever seen the counsellor despite a wish to do so; the general conclusion was that she was too 'afraid' of them to entertain a direct referral.

Equally, however, social work at Hospital Tranquillity was also under-utilised by patients and appeared to play a marginal and low status role in the daily activities of the hospital. Somewhat surprisingly, in view of its profile in community psychiatry elsewhere, no mention was made of the hospital's social work team as key players in future community-based services. In the other Asian regions, such as Hong Kong, social work is a crucial component in terms of smoothing the transition from hospital to successful community living, much as it has been in the UK (Pang *et al.*, 1997).

Predictably the role of social work at the hospital was seen exclusively in terms of 'bed clearing', a restrictive stereotype that can nonetheless be found in hospital institutions universally, and subject to orders by those higher up in the hierarchy (Barrett, 1996; Brian, 1986; Penhale, 2000). Because social work-type posts in Malaysia have to-date yet to be formally earmarked for qualified, university-trained social workers (Baba *et al.*, 2010), the two existing social work professionals at Tranquillity were heavily reliant on the second-hand guidance of the CPN team. The CPN attempted to outline their colleagues' duties, according to a nursing understanding of the social work remit, as unfortunately neither practising 'social worker' at that time had qualifications or a background in social work. Referrals therefore tended to concentrate purely on locating families of patients in order to effect discharges and skills. Social work skills therefore were dedicated towards essential detective work and subsequent negotiation to ensure that families took responsibility for the care of patients, as described in this account by a social worker.

> *Relatives move and the hospital cannot trace addresses. Some relatives run away from the patient, one mother left her son here for one month and said she would take him back when he was well. But when the patient was ready to go home the mother had gone, she had moved to X. So we have no choice but to send him back to the longhouse and hope the other residents look after him. I was angry with the mother, but also you can't blame her, because the patient was violent at home,*

asking for money and she was the only carer. But also she didn't control him or help him take his medication, didn't supervise him at all. Many families don't want to take relatives home, they don't see this as a hospital, a hospital where people are discharged – they see this as a place for crazy people to live. And they think the Government should take care of them.

Unfortunately, then the hospital plans for community-based services did not seem to incorporate a feasible alternative vision for patients other than that of continuing to live with relatives. This is a situation, which even in the context of the UK with its attendant supportive services and financial benefits, is described by one author as 'precarious, and contingent upon the good will of family members' (Hatfield *et al.*, 1992-3: 32-3). Given this situation the distinction, to quote Foucault, between 'care in the community and care by the community' remains somewhat clouded, with some tragic repercussions befalling patients whose families were clearly opposed to their presence (Foucault, 1976: 44). In one particular telling example, a social worker described a case where a multiply admitted man that I happened to know by sight, was discharged back to the care of his family, despite the fact that he was being kennelled in a stifling zinc-roofed cell in the garden. After one unsuccessful suicide attempt, which resulted in a readmission to Tranquillity, he was once again turned over to his relatives, where he finally succeeded in hanging himself. It is a rather telling indictment of social work assessments conducted at the hospital that although his home circumstances were reviewed, strangely enough they were not pronounced as clearly unsuitable for his needs.

Furthermore, in addition to their limited training, hospital social workers at Tranquillity were expected to act as autonomous hospital agents, independent from social services and effectively cut off from support from social work peers. Their ability to challenge their restrictive role and advocate on behalf of their clients, had they so wished to do, would therefore have been very limited, as was the time spent on the wards. Social work intervention was limited to a tight agenda, where no direct assessment of needs was carried out with clients, apart from a general home assessment. For the most part the social work team demonstrated a reluctance to engage with patients whose needs were largely unvarying and difficult to meet. Wards in turn were viewed as grim, unchangeable and depressing places, which were generally unnecessary to visit and so best avoided.

The views of medical officers

My contact with medical officers was much less frequent than those with nurses and medical assistants. Their presence on the wards were spasmodic, brief and business-like and therefore did not permit close observation over a period of time, and so I did not seek them out for some time until I had familiarised myself more fully with the world of patients and of nursing staff. When I did, I found that, with some notable exceptions, doctors of all ranks were approachable and some even took pleasure in adopting an instructive role. This pedagogic attitude however could take on the form of bullying behaviour, exemplified by the newcomer Dr Jerry, an overbearing and strangely antagonistic senior doctor who had already racked up a high level of unpopularity amongst the staff. I found it interesting that he took such a delight in baiting me by evading my own questions and instead posing others designed to highlight my ignorance. Apart from the fact that all such encounters represent grist to the researcher's mill, this was otherwise a frustrating and not very illuminating process, but evidently not entirely unusual, as Robin Brian (1986) notes of his own similar experience as a researcher in a sociological study of psychiatrists in Britain.

Doctors at Tranquillity are normally young male house officers governed by a couple of trained psychiatrists, which included the director himself. These house officers are in the business of acquiring a number of specialisms, of which psychiatry was only one and often far from the favourite. Like the majority of the nursing staff, serving doctors tended to regard their posting at Tranquillity as a temporary bond that increased their general medical experience and added to their marketable skills. Some, however, announced that they had little choice in terms of transfer and were here actively 'against their will'; a situation that one angry doctor denounced as a demoralising and counterproductive measure that necessarily impacted on the care of patients.

> We have internal politics about the level of staff, and OK I am not the best medical officer in the world, but some of the others are worse. It's a symptom of how sick things are here: people are transferred against their will, and unless you're really bad, for the Government's part they don't try to keep you happy, you try to keep them happy. If I am bad they won't sack me, if I am not happy, I quit. Other places if you don't do the job you lose the tender; here you don't lose the tender until you fall out of political favour.

In common with nurses and medical assistants, vocational commitments of doctors towards psychiatry as a discipline were not usual. This made Dr

Khairul's attitude all the more unusual in feeling that work in psychiatry was reasonably rewarding, an area 'where you can see progress in patients', but unattractive as a career if one stayed in Government-run posts due to the poor salary and career prospects. Consequently, however interesting he found psychiatry, he intended to leave the hospital and enter private general practice as soon as possible, where in fact the majority of the State's available psychiatrists were unfortunately already located.

Regardless of the expertise that in theory existed in the hospital, the dearth of alternative therapies, such as psychotherapeutic interventions, coupled with the discouraging conditions and attitudes operating at the hospital, made some doctors long to set up practice for a more stimulating and probably less challenging, fee-paying clientele. Hierarchies of treatment were obviously dependent upon the economic strata and purchasing power of categories of patient, as noted by Joop de Jong (2001), and this represented a notable and lamentable aspect of institutional life at Tranquillity.

> On a number of occasions I witnessed colleagues in Asia giving large amounts of drugs and electro-convulsive therapy (ECT) for a variety of diagnoses to low income patients, while reserving (psychoanalytic) psychotherapy for a small elite in a private practice (de Jong, 2001: 139).

Dr Fabian, unusually for a man, 'followed' his wife to Kuching, where she was fortunate in obtaining a more successful post than the one he held at Tranquillity. Dr Fabian was clearly unhappy in his work, regarding psychiatry in quite the opposite way to that of Dr Khairul as being an area where work was demoralising because progress was almost imperceptible. Along with his more enthusiastic colleague he saw it as a dead-end career and palpably yearned to escape. Additionally, and perhaps most importantly, he seemed very bothered by how medical colleagues regarded the work, which added to his general dissatisfaction and frustration.

> *There's a lot of stigma in being in a psychiatric hospital in Malaysia. Do you agree with me? And when you tell people, other doctors, you work at Hospital Tranquillity, they say, 'Oh, that place!' It's not easy to be here. Some people, even you know, doctors, seem to think that if you work here long enough you might become insane as well – it's contagious, sort of thing.*

The stigma of working at the hospital did not only impact on doctors but was a concern that nurses and medical assistants also acknowledged, as confided by one individual working on a male chronic ward:

I work here for the family's sake. But there is stigma working here. Other staff ask you where you work and .... they smile ... there is stigma working here. One time I didn't say where I worked, I'd say [substitutes a name]. Not many people want to work here.

Stigma was therefore regarded as the major enemy militating against community acceptance of people with mental illnesses, with the resulting assumptions that wards would continue to exist occupied by patients who were unlikely ever to be discharged. The prevailing perception amongst lower-ranking doctors and nursing staff conformed with Estroff's (1981) analysis that it was unrealistic to hope that the labelling and social discarding of patients would be prevented through the adoption of community-based services.

Prior to commencing fieldwork, although aware of stigma I had grossly underestimated the extent of this prejudice towards mental illness in this region. Staff accounts sharpened an otherwise vague appreciation of the issues at stake. Furthermore, prominent participants such as the former State Psychiatrist further enlightened me through his opinion that mental illness was regarded as being *more* stigmatising than leprosy, a frequently occurring disease in the region in the recent past. If Foucault employed this analogy as largely a symbolic motif, this individual by contrast pragmatically talked in shockingly literal terms (Foucault, 1965). Accordingly, staff indicated that working in a psychiatric hospital was perceived as not only stigmatising on a professional basis, but as psychologically and perhaps even morally hazardous in its insidious contagion.

Given personal agendas such as these, few house officers focused their attention on incipient plans towards community psychiatry. In the meantime dissent high in the ranks was articulated by Dr Jerry who disapproved of the entire endeavour and scathingly dismissed it as yet another tired example of post-colonialism paradigms inappropriately imposed on developing nations (Bhugra, 2001; Littlewood, 2001; McCulloch, 2001).

Dr J:	Community psychiatry is rubbish! I've told them that in Kuala Lumpur. It was all started by the British - and in Malaysia we have to copy *everything* Britain does, even if it's wrong!
Researcher:	What kind of model of care would you like to see instead?
Dr J:	Where you'd get large numbers of psychiatrists and trained staff, all trying to compete with each other and learning from each other. Instead of this situation where you get

> a psychiatrist here or there, doing as they please, with no
> one looking at what they do. This is the way other health
> practices are managed, like the Cardiac Centre in KL (Kuala
> Lumpur). This is where all the knowledge and technology
> is concentrated, and not just heart problems, most other
> medical specialities. We should be doing the same with
> psychiatry. It would be much better for the profession.
>
> *Researcher:*   And the patients?
>
> *Dr J:*   Them too.

Suman Fernando (2010: 113) is highly critical of the imposition of
psychiatric models on postcolonial nations, commenting on the pressure
of such countries to adopt Western-style community-care models, along
with a heavily pharmacological approach, that may not be 'suited to local
conditions'. Dr Jerry's scorn for the expertise of the former colonial master
and its ilk would therefore accord well with this critique. However, for those
who may adhere to a basic belief in community psychiatry, Dr Jerry's vision of
centralised services would represent a nightmare return to the vast asylums
of yesteryear on the pretext of improved service provision and psychiatric
excellence. Ironically, in reality this would barely move away from the
models of care that Dr Jerry regarded as defunct and exhausted, as well as
inappropriate for modern, independent Malaysia (Acharyya, 1996; Barham,
1992; Deva, 1992). Narratives, such as these, point to a continuing tension
that exists between ideologies that are predicated on polarised models of
care. These nonetheless retain a grip on values and practices influenced by
the West, but which are mutually incompatible (Campbell, 1996; Caplan
and Caplan, 2000; Forrester-Jones, 1985).

The abyss between the vision of community psychiatry and the realities
of maintaining an increasingly institutionalised and ageing population of
asylum patients, made it difficult for staff to make the required imaginative
leap towards alternative scenarios of community care. The focus of doctors
and nurses was therefore engaged in the daily business of maintaining order
and making at least token attempts to improve the lives of patients in their
care. The main fixation was with the immediate working environment and
daily interactions with colleagues in the course of undertaking duties.

In general, and understandably so, lower-status individuals such as
medical assistants and nurses were often uncomfortable about offering
comments on the behaviour and attitudes of higher-status staff, specifically
the doctors in charge. It was therefore highly problematic gathering
information on what nurses and medical assistants thought of doctors,

short of inferred nuance and veiled implication. On the other hand, doctors were more likely to feel able to comment on similar issues in relation to lower-status colleagues, with some reservations, although obviously wary of seeming to criticise those above them and hospital policies in general. Notably, among house officers disinterest and disillusion with work at the hospital seemed to be a dominant theme. These attitudes extended beyond their own particular circumstances and were directed to those further down the hierarchy as well. Often a dim view was taken of the quality of nursing care undertaken at the hospital. Some doctors in interview were quite scathing in their evaluation of their colleagues' work, but equally rather nervous of retaliation to open criticism that apparently both could be and had been rewarded by petty acts of revenge, both in and outside of the hospital setting. Most of these doctors had enjoyed a traditional training overseas in developed countries, such as Britain. During this time they had been embraced in a medical culture of agreed expectations and values that were apparently shaken upon their return home and particularly so in relation to their work at Tranquillity.

Well after all, I've lowered my expectations, haven't I. I mean I just don't expect ....I came back from 3 years overseas and .... Hey, when I start a job it's the nursing staff that teach me things, they look out for me, they know! But you can't expect that here. You just get, 'whatever you want doctor'. I mean there's nothing! You can't expect it. Developing nation! I don't know what's expected in Malaysia, I only know what's in this hospital. It has low calibre staff. Problem staff get dumped here - transferred here. By the time they end up here there's a problem, although obviously I'm not talking about everyone. The staff here are pretty institutionalised themselves.

The almost inevitable 'institutionalisation' that could be found amongst patients *and* staff alike was a common theme amongst doctors still undergoing adjustment to the hospital environment. This served to reinforce anxieties about their own circumstances and prospects whilst underscoring the need for more support and guidance from nursing colleagues, who under other circumstances were likely to be viewed as knowledgeable and trustworthy guides.

You find some (patients) in the chronic wards Male 2 and 3, lying under tables and things like that. Some have been here 15 to 20 years, longer! There's not a lot you can do with them. And the other staff, some nurses and MAs well they feel, that's what chronic patients are like. It's taken for granted that there's not much you can do to help them...Some of the nurses and MAs are quite good, the older ones are very good, but many of the nurses and even MAs have slacked off and compared to the general hospital not so well medically trained, they don't know what to do. They've gone rusty.

The subsequent effort involved in attempting to bring progress to the wards was raised as an arduous, difficult and indeed futile task in many cases, with the inertia of nursing staff opposing the authority of these 'new brooms'. The general view amongst new doctors was that too often any change that they initiated flew in the face of an entrenched attitude by nursing staff, as described in this account by a female doctor.

'You not only don't do what I want, you sabotage my treatment! Why don't I just give you a bucket of pills and let you do what you want!' Hey who cares? These are psychiatric patients. In this country if they die the family think 'good'. You've [directed to researcher] *seen the four chronic wards, they're abandoned people.*

Finally, while gender differences could be seen to play an important role in relation to nursing staff, this was not an area that could be adequately explored amongst serving doctors at the hospital. The unfortunate consequence of the scarcity of female doctors inevitably meant that in relation to the topic of work and careers insufficient gender-based analysis could be brought to bear upon the position of women and male doctors. It would be fair to say, however, that amongst doctors of both sexes and all ranks, very few regarded their post at Tranquillity as being other than a temporary and frustrating sojourn. Even for those with a commitment to mental health work their sights were set on opportunities elsewhere. Psychiatry at Tranquillity was accordingly seen to be an unrewarding business in terms of professional careers and working conditions; and for those intending to retain some interest in psychiatry, the traditionally lucrative business of private practice, rather than asylum management, was seen as by far the best personal option.

10
Reflections and conclusions

As with most, if not all, ethnographic studies, the final destination is never clear from the outset. Fieldwork, analysis and the writing-up of findings create a picture of organised industry to readers that in fact disguises the reality of the ethnographic journey which is far more fragmented, chaotic and exhilarating. While unlike the sanitised conditions under which the stereotypic quantitative natural scientist works, ethnographic research encounters with participants embroil the researcher in complex and multi-layered relationships that resonate long after fieldwork is over. There is therefore no cut-and-dried way of wrapping up ethnographic research and the 'mulling over' of experiences and dilemmas continue to colour the way one understands 'findings', even if the final interpretation may not metamorphose so very much over the years. In addition, of course, new issues continually emerge as the site of the study and the participants one knew change and generally move on. Distilling the essence of the study into a neat set of conclusions is therefore no easy task, but one that offers an important opportunity to reconsider initial discoveries and integrate these into some further observations and reflections.

The enduring nature of the asylum

When I first began work at Hospital Tranquillity, I consciously rejected the dubious role of being the omniscient, judgemental, foreign expert and was instead open to being impressed by how professionally this small hospital committed itself to the needs of its widespread, multicultural community, in view of its somewhat limited resources. I remain impressed by how much is done for psychiatric patients and their families, given an ambitious agenda tied to an ambivalent political climate towards psychiatric services and patients. Furthermore, some of the staff I met were genuinely compassionate and skilled, having proved their personal commitment towards good standards of practice over the course of years, which must have been a difficult task as staff accounts make clear. Since spending so much time gathering the accounts of patient participants on the somewhat grim, if usually scrupulously scrubbed open wards, my dominant feelings are dismay at the amount of wasted potential harboured by the hospital system.

Patient accounts, for instance, record in often quite matter-of-fact ways the daily trials and humiliations imposed upon them by institutional rituals and routines that appear to have little rationale other than to impose a seemingly futile semblance of order and control, a discipline for discipline's sake approach. This is in addition to the more laudible attempt to create a meaningful structure out of interminable days that would otherwise lack virtually any texture or variety. The lives of long-stay patients, as well as those destined to become the next cohort, convey lasting impressions of lost opportunities and personal degradation in the long years sequestered behind walls. These accounts are as indicative of the need for change in contemporary Malaysian services, as embodied by Hospital Tranquillity, as they are evocative of traditional asylum care.

Over time, the force of what was seen and heard during time spent at the site convinced me that hospital life had in fact not changed very much from institutional practices that had in many places now been generally outmoded. Sadly at Hospital Tranquillity, despite certain attempts to modernise services, an attitude of disregard of civil rights and a lack of respect for user perspectives endured. Modernisation in this sense of the word referred largely to keeping abreast of the latest in medication regimes and forming expansion plans. Significantly, these were not visualised as improving by one iota the lives of those patients whose existence had been overshadowed by institutional care the longest. This group of patients was the dispensable generation, 'abandoned' not just by the community, but from any hope from their professional carers that they would experience change for the better in their lifetime.

Despite a more publicly friendly face for visitors, Hospital Tranquillity has remained a good example of the 'total institution'. Certainly, the conditions and descriptions of life in British Victorian psychiatric hospitals were not been so far removed from the daily workings of this contemporary hospital. In its spatial geography and social, as well as sexually segregated areas, the hospital is an example of the self-contained asylum. In this respect, the hospital acts as a contemporary and miniaturised version of the institutions typical of the nineteen century, which sought to impose social and gender normative values, in terms of physical geography and isolation from society. This is not to imply that treatment at Tranquillity is barbaric, that would be an unfair assertion, both untrue of the hospital and its staff, and a distortion of the best that the nineteenth century's institutional care sought to achieve, in intention at least, if not always in practice.

Thus men and women occupied separate facilities at Hospital Tranquillity and enjoyed no social interaction that was not heavily subject to custodial measures by staff, in keeping with traditional asylum practices in Europe. Furthermore, class differentials were demarcated through the differences in conditions, diet and freedom of patient access between the congested third class 'public' wards and the more liberal, infinitely more pleasant, sparsely populated 'private', fee-paying first and second class wards. The differences between the conditions of men and women patients on the wards were accordingly characterised by both gender and class distinctions.

Consequently, the asylum system was in fact very much alive and well in East Malaysia, and it is likely that this is not an anomaly nationally. Despite attempts to change affairs, whether concerted or half-hearted, it apparently seemed extremely difficult to relieve the otherwise unchanging face of institutional care with all its attendant miseries and privations. Yet, changes that are actively in the process of being offered, such as community-based psychiatry, hold an uncertain future. Although this offered one model of Western ideology attractive to the Government and to the upper hospital administration, staff perceptions all too frequently regarded it as an irrelevance, out-of-step with their views of psychiatric nursing and acceptance by the public. From the point of view of patient care, moves towards a community-based programme jarred with the current situation of a strictly professional, hierarchical and undemocratic power base: because the ideology behind this movement in the West has not been embraced, alongside the practical concept. However, equally it must be recognised that without the social infrastructure necessary to support community care - and indeed, as has been found in the West, even despite it – the psychiatric institution may arguably still function as a refuge from the neglect or abuse that may otherwise befall the vulnerable who are not willingly cared for outside. Fernando (2010), normally a scathing critic of the contemporary legacy of colonial psychiatry, offers a word of caution about idealising indigenised forms of care where these involve abusive practices, such as had been witnessed in South India, for instance. This caveat is reminiscent of a report by Jackson (2005) of the release of a mentally ill man in Zimbabwe who was chained to a tree for ten years by his own father, as the only means of control. Interestingly, this episode was framed by the Zimbabwe African National Union as a grand symbolic gesture of liberation from colonisation - and as a critique of colonial psychiatry.

Reform in terms of community psychiatry in Malaysia, evidently remains an anomalous situation therefore, unless it is eventually interpreted as staking a claim to form a new and indigenised psychiatric system for the community, and one that shares no common assumptions and ideologies to similar moves taking place in other industrialised nations. Since a Westernised ideology of care, together with its practice, has been traditionally accepted in Malaysia (as one can see from its history of colonial psychiatric services), to sever guiding principles from practices would be a radical departure from a retrospective trend towards replication of Western-type services, even when these have carried prejudicial views towards patients. However, this does not mean that such an evolution to indigenised psychiatry is not afoot, and, if established, this might well in future be seen as more appropriate for the care of regional populations than the systems currently in place. As yet, however, without further clarification of goals and intentions, such a development remains speculation only.

For patients themselves, the distinctions of care based upon gender, class and ethnicity cast doubt on how therapeutic the asylum, as a haven, can actually be; even if it offers some refuge from the pressures and dangers of the external world. Prejudice towards women at Tranquillity is clearly rife in institutional attitudes and practices, women being discriminated against at multiple levels in their daily existence. Due to the constraints of life in the hospital the reproduction of these patriarchal practices are refined in their most damaging forms. Oppression in terms of enforced and confined access makes literal and abject prisoners of women patients in particular. The repercussions of this are seen to impact on women at a variety of levels personally and socially, as well as in relation to work and health.

Furthermore, the subsuming of concepts of femininity, sexuality and fertility in relation to class distinctions serves to impose the heaviest set of restrictions on working-class, pre-menopausal women. While in terms of meaningful activity, apart from encouraging narcissistic preoccupations with stereotypic notions of Western female glamour, the pastime of most women patients has revolved solely around deeply exploitative and unskilled labour, masquerading as meaningful therapeutic work, as well as providing unpaid, general care-giving on the wards. Staff attitudes towards women with mental illness at Tranquillity are therefore fraught with connotations of deranged incompetence and wilful as well as wanton conduct. These time-worn caricatures and historical views of feminine madness are a far cry from the positions of power and equality usually associated with women of Southeast Asia. Thus the conditions and attitudes under which women patients at Tranquillity live demand further research of women's experiences, in relation to the psychiatric services in this region, in order to ascertain the extent of traditional discrimination towards hospitalised women service users.

In those areas where no gender difference could be specifically detected, the general professional attitude towards patients *per se* is deeply negative and once again, oppressive. The issue of medication, for example, raises more questions than answers. At Tranquillity, however, it is clear that medication issues impact heavily upon both sexes and reveal that, despite a rich tradition in indigenous and cross-cultural views of abnormal behaviour and aetiology, cultural interpretations make little impact on the dominant influence of a strict medical model. This lends credibility to arguments that psychiatry is a form of contemporary colonialism imposed by descendents of former subject nations upon fellow citizens. In consequence, strategies of resistance devised by patients hold no other import than that which would indicate a high level of individual sickness, deviance or obtuseness, or a combination of all three.

Furthermore, although the administration of ECT was beginning to be reviewed at the hospital in the 2000, up to that time it had played a dual role of being viewed as a normal medical procedure quelling problems in controlling patients on overcrowded wards. This kind of medical regime could easily be regarded as at least of doubtful practice; and is once again reminiscent of some of the worst abuses of the traditional asylum system, albeit one that has clear precedents in other countries. Overcrowding of course is a common feature of institutional life where compulsory detention is the norm, most notoriously in prison surroundings, and consequently the liberal use of lock-up sections are reminders that madness has invariably been associated in the public and professional mind with criminality.

Finally, if life for patients was far from being empowering or pleasant, staff respondents equally provided some interesting and indeed often disturbing accounts of a generally inhospitable working environment and the ensuing professional dissatisfaction. Due to the autonomous nature of wards, policy statements, such as those prescribing open wards, are not likely to be strictly followed. Rather they appear to be viewed by staff as operating in a permissive environment of staff interpretation in which practice often runs independently of policy, rather than influencing the latter. These attitudes therefore can translate into heavy paternalism and worse – a corrosive prejudice towards psychiatric patients, a notable aspect being the disfavouring of certain patients on ethnic grounds. The evidence from this study offers some clues regarding the predominance of Chinese patients and suggests once again an area of enormous potential for future research, ideally modelled on indigenous needs and interpretations.

To return to the experience of staff, this situation results in or exacerbates the shortfall of personnel at the hospital; and as such is strongly indicative of the stigma associated with working at a psychiatric hospital. This in turn leads to the use of non-voluntary and often temporary transfers of staff, many of whom are inexperienced or disinterested in psychiatric care, and often reluctant to find themselves posted to a psychiatric institutional setting in the first place. The outcome of such attitudes and practices results inexorably in significant levels of demoralisation and apathy among staff, leading to a high turn-over. This demotivating tendency helps to create a culture of indifference and in the more severe cases, gives rise to staff prejudice towards and fear of their charges. Such an environment of anxiety and defensiveness creates difficult and unpleasant working conditions for staff that are not easily subject to positive change.

The enormous stigma extended to psychiatric patients, particularly women, coupled with the top-down, patriarchal structure of Malaysian society weigh heavily against the logical evolution towards the greater empowerment of service users. I have no doubt, however, that this, as is happening with people with disabilities nationally, will eventually occur; although the form that will take may well be very different from that which has created the consumer/service user landscape in the West. Psychiatric service users, in all likelihood with the help of committed professionals, may well transform the face of psychiatric services in Malaysian society. My hope is that the words and wisdom of the participants in this study will be viewed as having made a small but vital contribution to this vision, by reminding us of how much society loses when medical labels result in such drastic social exclusion and scapegoating of troubled individuals. The compelling descriptions by patient participants inform us that their personal potential has been cruelly lopped and often far more through social rejection and mandatory detention for years on end than through the progress of illness. Thus it is that patients cannot satisfactorily pursuing self-insight and personal healing without the risk of being further judged as pathologically sick. These powerful drives towards wholeness, which have been recorded here, are prevented from being better synthesised at cognitive and emotional levels. This regrettably leads to further losses to the community, where otherwise such individuals could be a valuable source of help and advice to others. In other countries, this has worked to form the basis of a public educational and advocacy role that many current and ex-psychiatric service users have willingly undertaken. Having made a perilous and often lonely odyssey these people have returned to speak of their experiences and in so doing support others, being duly enriched in the self-knowledge that such descents bestow.

Finally, in reference to the very different journey of the professional ethnographer, the conclusion of work normally heralds the severing of meaningful fieldwork relationships with departure from the field, although not disengagement with the issues the study has raised. However well this departure is planned in theory, there is often a level of angst involved, relating to the disquieting feeling that maybe having plundered one's participants of their precious narratives the metaphorical midnight train out of town will shortly be leapt upon for new terrain and adventures. This anxiety was especially heightened for me in relation to this study, where I could not easily explain to all my patient participants the reasons for my departure. My fear was that for many of these people my absence from the site could have been regarded as a further betrayal, over and above the many that they had experienced on the path to permanent patient-hood.

In the end, I did manage to bid a personal farewell to all my closest contacts, shaking many a gnarled hand in the process. A large number of these participants were destined to remain behind at the hospital for years, with few hopes that they too would one day leave permanently. I recognise with sadness that for these individuals they may have been given the choice to speak of their lives at the hospital, which they often did with great generosity of spirit, but not to leave, as I had always been free to do.

References

Acharyya, S., 1996. Practicing cultural psychiatry: the doctor's dilemma. *In*: Heller, T., Reynolds, J., Gomm, R., Muston, R. and Pattison, S. eds. *Mental Health Matters*. Houndsmill, Basingstoke. The Open University/Macmillan, pp. 339-345.

Acton, M.,1990. Violence and mental illness: Some implications for social workers *Practice*, 4 (4), 285-296.

Agar, M.,1996. *The Professional Stranger*, 2nd Edition. San Diego: Academic Press

Alcott, L., 1991. The problem of speaking for others, *Cultural Critique*. 1991- 1992, Winter, 2-31.

Alexander, F.G. and Selesnick, S.T., 1967. *The History of Psychiatry*. London: George Allen & Unwin.

Appell, L.W.R., 1991. Sex role symmetry among the Rungus of Sabah. *In*: Sutlive, V. H., ed. *Female and Male in Borneo: Contributions and Challenges to Gender Studies*. Shanghai, VA: Borneo Research Council Monograph, pp. 1-56.

Ardener, S., 1995. The fieldwork experience. *In*: Ellen, R.F., ed. *Ethnographic Research: A Guide to General Conduct*. London/San Diego: Academic Press, pp. 63-87.

Ashencaen Crabtree, S., 1999a. Stigma and exclusion: Implications for community psychiatric services in Sarawak, Malaysia, *Asia Pacific Journal of Social Work International Journal*, 9 (1), 114-126.

Ashencaen Crabtree, S., 1999b. Teaching anti-discriminatory practice in Malaysia, *Social Work Education International Journal*. 18 (3), 247-255.

Ashencaen Crabtree, S. and Baba, I., 2001. Islamic perspectives in social work education: implications for teaching and practice, *Social Work Education*. 20 (4), 469-481.

Ashencaen Crabtree, S. and Chong, G., 2000. Mental Health and Citizenship in Malaysia, *International Social* Work, 43 (2) April, 217-226.

Ashencaen Crabtree, S. and Chong, G., 1999. Psychiatric outreach work in Sarawak, Malaysia, *Breakthrough International Journal*. 2 (4), 49-60.

Asher, R.M. and Fine, G.A., 1991. Fragile ties: Shaping research relationships with women married to alcoholics. *In*: Shaffir, W.B. and Stebbins, R. A., eds. *Experiencing Fieldwork*. Newbury Park, C.A./ London: Sage Publications, pp.196-206

Aull Davies, C., 1999. *Reflexive Ethnography*. London/New York: Routledge.

Aunger, R., 1995. On Ethnography, Storytelling or Science? *Current Anthropologist,* 36 (1), 97-114.

Baba, I., Ashencaen Crabtree, S. and Parker, J., 2010. Future indicative, past imperfect: a cross-cultural comparison of social work education in Malaysia and England. In: Stanley, S., ed. *Social Work Education in Countries of the East: Issues and Challenges.* NY: Nova Publishers, pp. 279-301.

Baba, I., 1992. Social work - An effort towards building a caring society. *In:* Sin, C.K. and Salleh, I.M., eds. *Caring Society: Emerging Issues and Future Directions.* Malaysia: Institute of Strategic and International Studies.

Bailey, C.A., 1996. *A Guide to Field Research.* Thousand Islands, California: Pine Forge Press.

Bannister, P., 1999. Observation. *In:* Bannister, P., Parker, I.., Parker, I., Taylor, M. and Tindall, C., eds. *Qualitative Methods in Psychology, A Research Guide.* Buckingham: Open University Press, 17-33.

Barham, P., 1992. *Closing the Asylum.* London: Penguin Books.

Barham, P. and Hayward, R., 1996. The lives of 'users'. *In:* Heller, T., Reynolds, J., Gomm, R., Muston, R. and Pattison, S. eds. *Mental Health Matters.* Houndsmill, Basingstoke. The Open University/Macmillan, pp. 226-237.

Baron, C., 1987. *Asylum to Anarchy.* London: Free Association Books.

Barnes, M. and Bowl, R., 2001. *Taking Over the Asylum.* Basingstoke: Palgrave.

Barrett, R.J. (1993) 'Performance, Effectiveness and the Iban Manang', in R.L. Winzeler (Ed) *The Seen and the Unseen: Shamanism, Mediumship and Possession in Borneo'.* Virginia, USA: Ashley Printing Services

Barrett, R.J., 1996. *The Psychiatric Team and the Social Definition of Schizophrenia: An Anthropological Study of Person and Illness.* Cambridge/New York: Cambridge University Press.

Barrett, J., 1997. Cultural formulation of psychiatric diagnosis: *Sakit Gila* in an Iban longhouse: chronic schizophrenia, *Culture, Medicine and Psychiatry,* 21, 365-379.

Beasley, C., 1999. *What is Feminism?* London: Sage Publications.

Bell, D., 1993. Introduction 1. The Context'. *In:* Bell, D. and Caplan, P., eds. *Gendered Fields: Women, Men & Ethnography.* London: Routledge, pp. 1-18.

Bell, J., 1996. Label removed but scar remains. *In:* Read, J. and Reynolds, J., ed. *Speaking Our Minds: An Anthology of Personal Experiences of Mental Distress and Its Consequences.* Houndsmill, Basingstoke/The Open University/ MacMillan Press Ltd, pp. 105-108

Bentelspacher, C.E et al., 1994. Coping and adaptation patterns among Chinese, Indian & Malay families caring for a mentally ill relative, *Families in Society: The Journal of Contemporary Human Services,* May, 287-294.

Beresford, P. and Croft, S., 1993. *Citizen Involvement: A Practical Guide for Change*. Basingstoke: MacMillan Press

Berg, BL. 2007. *Qualitative Research Methods for the Social Sciences*, 6th ed. Boston: Allyn & Bacon.

Bernstein, J., 1993. The shaman's destiny: symptoms, afflictions and the re-interpretation of illness among the Taman. *In*: Winzeler, R.L., ed. *The Seen and the Unseen: Shamanism, Mediumship and Possession in Borneo*. Virginia, USA: Ashley Printing Services, pp. 171-206.

Bhopal, K., 1997. *Gender, 'Race' and Patriarchy. A Study of South Asian Women*. Aldershot: Ashgate.

Bhugra, D., 1997. Setting up psychiatric services: Cross-cultural issues in planning and Delivery, *International Journal of Social Psychiatry*, Spring 43 (1), 1-16.

Bhugra, D., 2001. The colonized psyche: British influence on Indian psychiatry. *In*: Bhugra, D. and Littlewood, R., eds. *Colonialism and Psychiatry*. Oxford: Oxford University Press, pp. 46-76.

Black, B. J., 1988. *Work and Mental Illness; Transitions to Employment*. Baltimore: The John Hopkins University Press.

Blackwood, E., 1995. Senior Women, model mothers, and dutiful wives: Managing gender contradictions in a Minangkabau village. *In* : Onw, A. and Peletz, M.G., eds. *Bewitching Women, Pious Men: Gender and Body Politics in Southeast Asia*. Berkeley: University of California, pp.124-158.

Blanc-Szanton, C., 1990. Collision of Cultures. Historical Reformulations of Gender in the Lowland Visayas, Philippines. *In*: Monnig Atkinson, J. and Errington, S., eds. *Power & Difference: Gender in Island Southeast Asia*. Stanford California: Stanford University Press, pp. 345-383.

Bose, R., 1997. Psychiatry and the popular conception of possession among the Bangladeshis in London, *Journal of Social Psychiatry*, 43 (1), 1-16.

Bracken, P.J., 1999. Psychiatry, psychotherapy and the Irish in Britain, *Breakthrough*, 2 (4), 29-37.

Brian, R., 1986. *Reproducing Psychiatry. An Ethnographic Study of Entry to an Occupation*. Unpublished PhD Thesis. University College Cardiff.

Brewer, J.D., 1994. The ethnographic critique of ethnography, *Sociology*. 28 (1), 232- 236.

Brewer, J.D., 2000. *Ethnography*. Buckingham: Open University Press.

Burgess, R.G., 1995. *In the Field: An Introduction to Field Research*. London/New York: Routledge.

Burgess, R.G., 1991. Sponsors, gatekeepers, members, and friends: Access in educational settings. *In*: Shaffir, W.B. and Stebbins, R. A., eds. *Experiencing Fieldwork*. Newbury Park, C.A./ London: Sage Publications, pp. 43-52.. Busfield, J., 1986. *Managing Madness: Changing Ideas and Practice*. London: Hutchinson.

Burman, E.,1999. Feminist Research. *In*: Bannister, P. ed. *Qualitative Methods in Psychology, A Research Guide*: Buckingham: Open University Press.

Busfield, J., 1994. The female malady? Men, women and madness in nineteenth century Britain, *Sociology*, 28 (1), 259-277.

Busfield, J., 1996a. *Men, Women and Madness*. Houndsmill, Basingstoke: MacMillan Press.

Busfield, J., 1996b. Professionals, the state and the development of mental health policy. *In*: Heller, T., Reynolds, J., Gomm, R., Muston, R. and Pattison, S. eds. *Mental Health Matters*. Houndsmill, Basingstoke. The Open University/ Macmillan, pp. 134-142.

Butler, A. and Pritchard, C., 1983. *Social Work and Mental Illness*. London: Macmillan Press.

Campbell, P., 1996. The history of the user movement in the United Kingdom'. *In*: Heller, T., Reynolds, J., Gomm, R., Muston, R. and Pattison, S. eds. *Mental Health Matters*. Houndsmill, Basingstoke. The Open University/Macmillan, pp. 218-225.

Caplan, G. and Caplan, R., 2000. Principles of community psychiatry, *Community Mental Health Journal*, 36 (1), 7-24.

Caplan, P., 1993. Introduction 2. The Volume. *In*: Bell, D. and Caplan, P., eds. *Gendered Fields: Women, Men & Ethnography*. London: Routledge, pp. 19-27.

Carter, P., Everitt, A. and Hudson, A., 1992. .Malestream training? Women, feminism and social work education. *In*: Langan, M. and Day, L., eds.*Women, Oppression and Social Work*. London/New York: Routledge, pp. 112-128.

Chakraborty, A., 1991. Culture, colonialism and psychiatry, *Lancet*. 337 (8751), 1204- 1208.

Chesler, P., 1972. *Women and Madness*. New York: Doubleday.

Chesler, P., 1996. *Women and madness: The mental asylum*. *In*: Heller, T., Reynolds, J., Gomm, R., Muston, R. and Pattison, S. eds. *Mental Health Matters*. Houndsmill, Basingstoke. The Open University/Macmillan, pp. 46-53.

Chen, H.-S., 1995. Developments of mental health systems in China from the 1940s through the 1980s. *In*: Tsung-Yi Lin, Wen-Shing Tseng and Eng-Kung Yeh., eds. *Chinese Societies and Mental Health*. Hong Kong: Oxford University Press, pp. 315-325.

Chew, D., 1990. *Chinese Pioneers on the Sarawak Frontier*. Singapore: Oxford University Press.

Chiu, T.L., Tong, J.E. and Schmidt, K.E., 1972. A clinical and survey study of latah in Sarawak, Malaysia. *Psychological Medicine*. 2, 155-165.

Chi-Ying Chung, C.-Y. R., Walkey, F.H. and Bemak, F., 1997. A comparison of achievement and aspirations of New Zealand Chinese and European Students, *Journal of Cross-Cultural Psychology*. 28 (4), 481-489.

Chowdhry, G., 1995. Engendering Development? Women in Development (WID) in International Development Regimes. *In*: Parpart, J.L. and Marchand, M.H., eds. *Feminism Postmodernism Development*. London: Routledge, pp. 26-41.

Chua, L., 2007. Fixity and flux: Bidayuh (dis)engagements with the Malaysian ethnic system, *Ethnos*, 72(2), 262-288.

Clammer, J.R., 1987. Approaches to ethnographic research. *In*: Ellen, R.F., ed. *Ethnographic Research: A Guide to General Conduct*. London/San Diego: Academic Press., pp. 63-86.

Clark, D., 1996. *The Story of a Mental Hospital, Fulbourn 1858-1983)*. London: Process Press.

Cleary, M. and Eaton, P., 1992. *Borneo, Change and Development*. Singapore: Oxford University Press.

Clifford, J., 1986. Introduction: Partial Truths. *In*: Clifford, J. and G. E. Marcus, G.E., eds. *Writing Culture: The Poetics and Politics of Ethnography*. Berkeley, Los Angeles/London: University of California Press, pp. 1-26.

Clive, 1996. I've got memories here. *In*: Read, J. and Reynolds, J., eds. *Speaking Our Minds: An Anthology of Personal Experiences of Mental Distress and Its Consequences*. Houndsmill, Basingstoke: The Open University/ MacMillan Press Ltd, pp. 129-30.

Cogliati, M.G., Petri, S. and Pini, M.T., 1988. Gender in the Italian services. *In*: Ramon, S. and Giannichedda, M.G., eds. *Psychiatry in Transition: The British and Italian Experience*. London: Pluto Press, pp. 99-108.

Cohen, A., 1998. Mental health issues among the indigenous peoples of the world. *WAPR Bulletin*, Geneva: WHO.

Cohen, A., 1999. *The Mental Health of Indigenous Peoples: An International Overview*. Geneva: WHO. Colson, A.C., 1971. The Perception of Abnormality in a Malay Village. *In*: Tan, E.-S. and Wagner, N.N., eds. *Psychological Problems and Treatment in Malaysia*. Kuala Lumpur: University of Malaya Press, pp. 88-101.

Cooper, D., 1970. *Psychiatry and Anti-Psychiatry*. London: Granada Publishing Co.

Connell, R.W., 2005. *Masculinities*, 2nd ed. Berkeley, CA: University of California Press.

Crabtree, S.A., 2001. A multicultural montage: Perspectives from care- giving families in Sarawak. *In*: Haque, A., ed. *Mental Health Issues in Malaysia, Issues and Concerns*. Kuala Lumpur: University of Malaya Press, pp. 147-162.

Crabtree S. and Chong, G., 2001. Standing at the crossroads: Mental health in Malaysia since Independence. *In*: Haque, A., ed. *Mental Health Issues in Malaysia, Issues and Concerns*. Kuala Lumpur: University of Malaya Press, pp. 21-34.

Davison, J. and Sutlive, V., 1991. The Children of *Nising*: Images of headhunting and male sexuality in Iban ritual and oral literature. *In*: Sutlive, V. H., ed. *Female and Male in Borneo: Contributions and Challenges to Gender Studies*. Shanghai, VA: Borneo Research Council Monograph, pp. 153-230

Day, L., 1992. Women and oppression: race, class and gender. *In*: Langan, M. and Day, L., eds.*Women, Oppression and Social Work*. London/New York: Routledge, pp.12-31.

DeLaine, M., 1997. *Ethnography: Theory and Applications in Health Research*. Sydney: Maclennan and Petty.

Denzin, N.K. 1997. *Interpretative Ethnography*. Thousand Oaks/London: Sage Publications.

Denzin, N.K and Lincoln, Y.S., 1995. Transforming qualitative research methods: is it A revolution?, *New Ethnographies*, October, 349 –356.

Department of Statistics., 1991. *General Report of the Population Census of Malaysia 1991*. Volume 2. Kuala Lumpur: Department of Statistics.

Desjarlais, R., 1996. The office of reason: On the politics of language and agency in a shelter for 'the homeless mentally ill, *American Ethnologist*, 23(4), 880-900.

Deva, M.P., 2004. Malaysia mental health country profile, *International Review of Psychiatry*, 16(1-2), 167-176.

Deva, M.P., 1992. Psychiatry and mental health in Malaysia: current state and future Directions. *In*: Sin, C.K. and Salleh, I.M., eds. *Caring Society: Emerging Issues and Future Directions*. Malaysia: Institute of Strategic and International Studies.

Deva, M.P., 1995. Medicine in Malaysia: Psychiatry, *Medical Journal of Malaysia*, 50, Supp-A, 570.

De Jong, J., 2001. Remnants of the colonial past: The difference in outcome of mental disorder in high- and Low-Income Countries. *In*: Bhugra, D. and Littlewood, R., eds. *Colonialism and Psychiatry*. Oxford: Oxford University Press, pp. 131-167.

Diaz-Canej, A. and Johnson, S., 2004.The views and experiences of severely mentally ill mothers – a qualitative study. *Social Psychiatry and Psychiatric Epidemiology*, 36(6), 472-82.

Dominelli, L., 1992. More than a method: feminist social work. *In*: K. Campbell, K., ed. *Critical Feminism: Argument in the Disciplines*. Buckingham: Open University Press, pp. 83-106.

Emerson, R.M., Fretz, R.I. and Shawm L.L., 1995. *Writing Ethnographic Fieldnotes*. Chicago/London: University of Chicago Press.

Erlandson, D.A., Harris, E.L., Skipper, B.L. and Allen, S.D., 1993. *Doing Naturalistic Inquiry: A Guide to Methods*. Newbury Park/London: Sage Publications.

210

Ernst, W., 2010. *Mad Tales From the Raj: Colonial psychiatry in South Asia, 1800-58*. London: Anthem Press.

Errington, S., 1990. Recasting sex, gender, and power. A theoretical and regional Overview. In: Atkinson, J.M. and Shelly Errington, S., eds. *Power and Difference: Gender in Island Southeast Asia*. Stanford California: Stanford University Press, pp. 1-58.

Estroff, S.E. , 1985. *Making It Crazy: An Ethnography of Psychiatric Clients in an American Community*. California: University of California Press.

Everitt, A., Hardiker, P., Littlewood, J. and Mullender, A., 1992. *Applied Research for Better Practice*. Houndsmill, Basingstoke: MacMillan Press Ltd/BASW.

Fabian, J., 1995. Ethnographic misunderstanding and the perils of context, *American Anthropologist*, 97 (1), 41-50.

Fadiman, A., 1997. *The Spirit Catches You and You Fall Down*. New York: Farrar, Strauss & Giroux.

Fallot, R.D., 2001. Spirituality and religion in psychiatric rehabilitation and recovery from mental illness, *International Review of Psychiatry*, 13 (2), 110-117.

Fennell, P., 1996. *Treatment Without Consent*. London/New York: Routledge.

Fernando, S., 2010. *Mental Health, Race and Culture*, 3rd ed. Houndsmill, Basingstoke: Macmillan Palgrave.

Fernando, S., 1995. *Mental Health in a Multi Ethnic Society*. London: Routledge.

Fernando, S., 1999. Ethnicity and mental health. *In*: Ulas, M. and Connor, A., eds. *Mental Health and Social Work*. London: Jessica Kingsley, pp. 119-142.

Fernando, S., Ndegwa, D. and Wilson, M., 2005. *Forensic Psychiatry, Race and Culture*. London/New York: Routledge.

Fetterman, D.M., 1991. A walk through the wilderness: Learning to find your way. *In*: Shaffir, W.B. and Stebbins, R. A., eds. *Experiencing Fieldwork*. Newbury Park, C.A./ London: Sage Publications, pp. 83-86.

Fidler, R.C., 1993. Spirit possession and exculpation: The Chinese of Sarawak. *In*: Winzeler, R.L., ed. (Ed) *The Seen and the Unseen: Shamanism, Mediumship and Possession in Borneo*. Virginia, USA: Ashley Printing Services, pp. 207-234.

Forrester-Jones, R., 1995. One Step to Freedom? An Applied Social Network and Ethnographic Study of People with Long-Term Mental health problems Resettled from Hospital in the Community. Unpublished PhD Thesis. *University of Wales Bangor*.

Foucault, M., 1965. *Madness and Civilization*. Cambridge: Cambridge University Press.

Foucault, M., 1976a. *Mental Illness and Psychology*. New York: Harper & Row.

Foucault, M., 1976b. *The Will to Knowledge: The History of Sexuality: 1*. London: Penguin Books.

Gabe, J., 1996. The history of tranquilliser use. *In*: Heller, T., Reynolds, J., Gomm, R., Muston, R. and Pattison, S., eds. *Mental Health Matters*. Houndsmill, Basingstoke. The Open University/Macmillan, pp. 186-195.

Gearing, J., 1995. Fear and loving in the West Indies: research from the heart (as well as the head. *In*: D. Kulick, D. and M. Wilson, M., eds. *Taboo: Sex, identity and erotic subjectivity in anthropological fieldwork*. London: Routledge, pp. 186-218.

Geller, J. L. and Harris, M., 1994. *Women of the Asylum*. New York: Anchor Books.

Gelsthorpe, L., 1992. Response to Martyn Hammersley's paper 'On feminist Methodology', *Sociology*, 26 (2) May, 213-218.

Gittins, D., 1998. *Madness in its place: Narratives of Severalls Hospital, 1913-1997*. London: Routledge.

Glick, P.B., 1998. Producing data. *In*: Ellen, R.F., ed. *Ethnographic Research: A Guide to General Conduct*. London/San Diego: Academic Press, pp. 213-294.

Goffman, E., 1968. The Mental Patient: Studies in the Sociology of Deviance. *In*: Spitzer, S.P. and Denzin, N.K., eds. *The Mental Patient: Studies in the Sociology of Deviance*. New York: McGraw-Hill Book Co., pp. 486-

Goffman, E., 1991. *Asylums: Essays on the social situation of mental patients and other inmates*. London: Penguin Books.

Goffman, E., 1993. The moral career of the mental patient. *In*: Pontell, H.N., ed. *Social Deviance: Readings in Theory and Research*. New Jersey: Prentice-Hall Inc.

Goldberg, A., 1999. *Sex, Religion and the Marking of Modern Madness*. Oxford/N.Y.: Oxford University Press.

Goldberg, D., Mubbashar, M. and Mubbashar, S., 2000. Development in mental health services – a world view. *International Review of Psychiatry*, 12, 240-248.

Goode, E., 1993. On behalf of labelling theory. *In*: Pontell, H.N., ed. *Social Deviance: Readings in Theory and Research*. New Jersey: Prentice-Hall Inc.

Gomm, R., 1996. Reversing deviancy. *In*: Heller, T., Reynolds, J., Gomm, R., Muston, R. and Pattison, S. eds. *Mental Health Matters*. Houndsmill, Basingstoke. The Open University/Macmillan, pp. 79-86.

Gostin, L., 1986. *Institutions Observed*. London: King's Fund.

Greasley, P., Chiu, L.F. and Gartland, M., 2001. The Concept of Spiritual Care in Mental Health Nursing. *Journal of Advanced Nursing*. 33 (5), 629-638.

Gullick, J.M., 1987. *Malay Society in the Late Nineteenth Century: The Beginnings of Change*. Singapore: Oxford University Press.

Gurney, J.N., 1991. Female researchers in male-dominated settings: Implications for short-term versus long-term research. *In*: Shaffir, W.B. and Stebbins, R. A., eds. *Experiencing Fieldwork*. Newbury Park, C.A./ London: Sage

Publications, pp. 53-61.

Gwee A.L., 1971. Traditional Chinese methods of mental treatment. *In*: Tan, E.-S. and Wagner, N.N., eds. *Psychological Problems and Treatment in Malaysia*. Kuala Lumpur: University of Malaya Press, pp. 102-

Halson, J., 1992. *Sexual Harassment, Oppression and Resistance: A Feminist Ethnography of Some Young People at Henry James School*. Unpublished PhD Thesis. University of Warwick.

Hammersley, M and Atkinson, P., 2010. *Ethnography: Principles in Practice*, 3rd ed. London: Routledge.

Hammersley, M and Atkinson, P., 1983. *Ethnography: Principles in Practice*. London/ New York: Tavistock Publishers.

Hammersley, M., 1990a. *Reading Ethnographic Research: A Critical Guide*. London: Longman.

Hammersley, M., 1990b. *What's Wrong With Ethnography*. London: Routledge.

Hammersely, M., 1992. On Feminist Methodology, *Sociology*. 26 (2) May, 187-206.

Hammersley, M., 2000. *Taking Sides in Social Research*. London: Routledge.

Harding, S., 1987. 'The Method Question'. *Hypatia*. 2 (3): 19-35.

Hatfield, B., Huxley, P. and Mohamad, H. 1992-3. The support networks of people with severe, long-term mental health problems, *Practice*, 6 (1), 25-40.

Hatta, S.M., 1996. A Malay crosscultural worldview and forensic review of amok, *Australian and New Zealand Journal of Psychiatry*, 30, 505-510.

Helman, C.G., 1984. *Culture, Health and Illness*. Oxford: Butterworth-Heineman:

Herzlich, C., 1995. Modern illness and the quest for meaning. Illness as a social Signifier. *In*: Augee, M. and Hertzlich, C., eds. *The Meaning of Illness Anthropology, History & Sociology*. Luxembourg: Harwood Academic Publishers, pp. 151-173.

Hester, M., 1994. Violence against social services staff: A gendered issue. *In*: Lupton, C. and Gillespie, T., eds. *Working with Violence*. Houndsmill, Basingstoke: Macmillan Press., pp. 153-169.

Hew, C. S., 1999. *Change, Continuity and Contradictions: Bidayuh Women, Migration. Wage Work and Family in Kuching, Malaysia*. Unpublished PhD Thesis. RMIT.

Hew, C.S., 2003. The Impact of Urbanization on Family Structure: The Experience of Sarawak, Malaysia, *SOJOURN*, 18 (1), 89-109.

Homan, R., 1991. *The Ethics of Social Research*. London/New York: Longman.

Higgins, R. and Hurst, K., 1999. *Psychiatric Nursing Revisited*. London: Whurr Publishers Ltd.

Hirsch, E. and Olson, G.A., 1995. Starting from Marginalized Lives: A Conversation with Sandra Harding. In: Olson G. A. and Hirsch, E., eds. *Women Writing Culture*. New York: State University of New York Press.

Holland, S., 1996. Developing a bridge to women's social action. In: Heller, T., Reynolds, J., Gomm, R., Muston, R. and Pattison, S. eds. *Mental Health Matters*. Houndsmill, Basingstoke. The Open University/Macmillan, pp. 304-308.

Homan, R., 1991. *The Ethics of Social Research*. London/New York: Longman.

Howard, N.C., McMinn, M.R., Bissell, L.D., Fairies, S.R. and VanMeter, J.B., 2000. Spiritual directors and clinical psychologists: A comparison of mental health and spiritual values. *Journal of Psychiatry and Theology*, 28 (4), 308-320.

Hudson, B., 1982. *Social Work with Psychiatric Patients*. London: MacMillan Press.

Humholtz, C., 1991. *Through Central Borneo*. Oxford: Oxford University Press.

Hustheesing, O. K., 1993. Facework of a female elder in a Lisu field, Thailand. In: Bell, D. and Caplan, P. *Gendererd Fields: Women, Men and Ethnography*. London/New York: Routledge, pp. 93-102.

Ijaz Gilani, A., Ijaz Gilani, U., Murtaza Kasi, P. And Murad Musa, K., 2005. Psychiatric health laws in Pakistan: From lunacy to mental health, *PLoS Medicine*, 2(1), 1105-1109.

Jablensky, A., 1995. Diagnosis and classification in a developing country. *Malaysian Journal of Psychiatry*, 3(1), 1-8.

Jackson, L., 2005. *Surfacing Up: Psychiatry and social order in colonial Zimbabwe*. New York: Cornell University Press.

Jamison, K.J., 1996. *An Unquiet Mind*. London: Picador.

Jane., 1996. I Want to Become Part of My Family Again. In: Read, J. and Reynolds, J., eds. *Speaking Our Minds: An Anthology of Personal Experiences of Mental Distress and Its Consequences*. Houndsmill, Basingstoke: The Open University/ MacMillan Press Ltd, pp. 111-115.

Jehom, W.J., 2001. The Bidayuh and being "Bidayuh" in Sarawak, *The Third Malaysian Studies Conference*, UKM Bangi. 6-8th August, 2001.

Jones, K., 1993. *Asylums and After*. London: The Athlone Press.

Jones, L., 1996. George III and the changing views of madness. In: Heller, T, Reynolds, J., Gomm, R., Muston, R. and Pattison, S. eds. *Mental Health Matters*. Houndsmill, Basingstoke. The Open University/Macmillan, pp. 121-135.

Karim, W. J., 1995. Bilateralism and gender in Southeast Asia. In: W. J. Karim, W. J., ed. *'Male' and 'Female' in developing Southeast Asia*. Oxford: Berg Publishers, pp. 11-34.

Kedit, P., 1991. 'Meanwhile Back Home...': Bejalai and their effects on Iban men and women. In: Sutlive, V. H., ed. *Female and Male in Borneo: Contributions and Challenges to Gender Studies*. Shanghai, VA: Borneo Research Council Monograph, pp. 295-316.

Keller, R., 2001. Madness and colonization: Psychiatry in the British and French empires, 1800-1962, *Journal of Social History,* Winter, 2001, 295-326.

Keller, R.C., 2007. Taking science to the colonies: Psychiatric innovation in France and North Africa. *In:* Mahone S. and Vaughan, M., eds. *Psychiatry and Empire.* Houndsmill, Basingstoke: Palgrave Macmillan, pp. 17-40.

Kelly, L., Burton, S. and Regan L., 1994. Researching women's lives or studying women's oppression? Reflections on What Constitutes Feminist Research. *In:* Maynard, M. and Purvis, J., eds. *Researching Women's Lives from a Feminist Perspective.* London: Taylor & Francis, pp. 27-48.

Kesey, K., 1962. *One Flew Over the Cuckoo's Nest.* New York: The New American Library Inc.

Khanna, R., 2003. *Dark Continents.* Durham/London: Duke University Press.

Kheng, C.B., 2003. Ethnicity, politics, and history textbook controversies in Malaysia. American Asian Review, XXI (4), 229-253.

Kielar, W., 1980. *Anus Mundi, Five Years in Auschwitz.* Harmondsworth, Middlesex: Penguin Books.

Kleinman, A., 1995. *Writing and the Margin.* Berkeley, CA.: University of California Press.

Kleinman, A., 1988a. *The Illness Narratives. Suffering, Healing and the Human Condition.* USA: Basic Books.

Kleinman, A., 1988b. *Rethinking Psychiatry: From Cultural Category to Personal Experience.* New York: The Free Press.

Kleinman, A., 1980. *Patients and Healers in the Context of Culture.* Berkeley, CA.: University of California Press.

Kleinman, A. and Gale, J. L., 1982. Patients treated by physicians and folk healers: A comparative outcome study in Taiwan, *Culture, Medicine and Psychiatry.* 6, 405 - 423.

Kleinman, A. and Kleinman, J., 1999. The transformation of everyday social experience: What a mental and social health perspective reveals about Chinese communities under global and local change, *Culture, Medicine and Psychiatry,* 23, 7-24.

Kleinman, A. and Kleinman, J., 1995. Remembering the cultural revolution: Alienating pains and the pain of alienation/transformation. *In:* Tsung-Yi Lin, Wen-Shing Tseng and Eng-Kung Yeh., eds. *Chinese Societies and Mental Health.* Hong Kong: Oxford University Press, pp. 141-155.

Kleinman, A. and Song, L.H., 1979. Why do indigenous practitioners successfully heal?, *Social Science and Medicine,* 130, 7-26.

Kleinman, S., 1991. Field-workers' feelings: What we feel, who we are, how we analyze. *In:* Shaffir, W.B. and Stebbins, R. A., eds. *Experiencing Fieldwork.* Newbury Park, C.A./ London: Sage Publications, pp. 184-195.

Knapen, H., 1997. Epidemics, droughts, and other uncertainties in Southeast Borneo during the eighteenth and nineteenth centuries. *In*: Boomgard, P., ed. *Paper Landscapes*. Leiden: KITLV Press, pp. 121-52

Knapen, H., 1998. Lethal diseases in the history of Borneo: mortality and the interplay between disease environment and human geography. *In*: King, V., ed. *Environmental Challenges in South-East Asia*. Richmond, Surrey: Curzon Press, pp. 69-94.

Kraepelin, E., 1962. *One Hundred Years of Psychiatry*. London: Peter Owen.

Kromm, J.E., 1994. The Feminization of madness in visual representation, *Feminist Studies*, 20 (3), 507-535.

Laderman, C., 1992. Malay Medicine, Malay Person. *In*: Nichler, M., ed. (Ed). *Anthropological Approaches to the Study of Ethnomedicine*. Amersterdam: Gordon & Breech Scientific Publishers, pp. 191-206

Laderman, C., 1996. The poetics of healing in Malay shamanistic performances. In: Laderman, C. and Roseman, M., eds. *The Performance of Healing*. New York/London: Routledge, pp.115-142.

Laderman, C., 1997. The embodiment of symbols and the acculturation of the anthropologist. *In*: Csordas, T.J.., ed. *Embodiment and Experience: The Existential Ground of Culture and Self*. Cambridge: Cambridge University Press, p. 183.

Laing, J., 1996. Leaving Carstairs. *In*: Read, J. and Reynolds, J., eds. *Speaking Our Minds: An Anthology of Personal Experiences of Mental Distress and Its Consequences'*. Houndsmill, Basingstoke: The Open University/MacMillan Press, pp. 95-99.

Lau, K.K. and Hardin, S., 1996. Community psychiatric nursing: An evaluation of schizophrenic patients in the first 3 years, *Medical Journal of Malaysia*, 51 (2), 242-254.

Leckie, J., 2007. Unsettled minds: gender and settling madness in Fiji. In: Mahone, S. and Vaughan, M. eds. *Psychiatry and Empire*. Houndsmill, Basingstoke: Palgrave Macmillan.

Lee, R.M., 1993. *Doing Research on Sensitive Topics*. London/Newbury Park: Sage Publications:

Levi, P., 1990. *If This is a Man*. London: Abacus.

Leibrich, J., 2002. Making Space: Spirituality and mental health, *Mental health, Religion & Culture*, 5 (2), 143-162.

Leighton, A. H. and Murphy, J.M., 1966. Cross-cultural psychiatry. In Murphy, L.J.M. and eighton, A.H., eds. *Approaches to Cross-Cultural Psychiatry*. Ithaca, N.Y: Cornell University Press, pp. 3-20.

Lefley, H., 1990. Rehabilitation in mental illness: Insights from other cultures, *Psychosocial Rehabilitation Journal*, 14 (1) July, 5-12.

Lemert, E.M., 1993a. Primary and secondary deviance. *In*: Pontell, H.N., ed. (Ed), *Social Deviance: Readings in Theory and Research*. New Jersey: Prentice-Hall.

Lemert, E.M., 1993b. Paranoia and the dynamics of exclusion. *In*: Pontell, H.N., ed. (Ed), *Social Deviance: Readings in Theory and Research*. New Jersey: Prentice-Hall Inc., pp. 418-

Lewis, I.M., 1995. *Ecstatic Religion: A Study of Shamanism and Spirit Possession*. London: Routledge.

Lewis, J., 1996. A review of prayer within the role of the holistic nurse, *Journal of Holistic Nursing*, 14 (4), 308.

Ling, H.K., 2007. *Indigenising Social Work: Research and practice in Sarawak*. Selangor: Strategic Information and Research Development Centre

Littlewood, R., 1991. From Disease to illness and back again, *Lancet*, 337 (8748), April, 10-13.

Littlewood, R., 2001. Colonialism and Psychiatry. *In*: Bhugra, D. and Littlewood, R., eds. *Colonialism and Psychiatry*. Oxford: Oxford University Press.

Littlewood, R. and Lipsedge M., 1989. *Aliens and Alienists*. London: Unwin Hyman.

Lis, C. and Soly, H., 1996. *Disordered Lives*. Cambridge: Polity Press.

Locke, K., 1996. Rewriting *The Discovery of Grounded Theory* after 25 Years, *Journal of Management Inquiry*, 5 (3) Sept, 239-245.

Loustaunau, H., 1989. An ethnomedical perspective of Ango-American psychiatry, *American Journal of Psychiatry*, 146 (5), 588-260.

Loustaunau, M.O. and Sobo, E.J., 1997. *The Cultural Context of Health, Illness and Medicine*. Westport, Connecticut/London: Bergin and Garvey.

Luchins, A., 1989. Moral treatment in asylums and general hospital in nineteenth century America, *Journal of Psychology*,123 (6), 585-607

Lützén, K., 1996. Research in psychiatric settings: Some ethical issues. *In*: De Raeve, L., ed. *Nursing Research: An Ethical and Legal Appraisal*. London: Ballière Tindall, pp. 71-84.

Lyons, L., 1999. Re-telling 'us: Displacing the white feminist subject as knower. Conference Paper. Workshop on Southeast Asian Women. Monash University: Melbourne.

Macintyre, M., 1993. Fictive kinship or mistaken identity? Fieldwork in Tubetube Island, Papua, New Guinea. *In*: Bell, D. and Caplan, P., eds. *Gendered Fields: Women, Men & Ethnography*. London: Routledge, pp. 44-62.

Manderson, L., 1996. *Sickness and the State, Health & Illness in Colonial Malaya 1870-1940*. Hong Kong: Cambridge University Press.

Marchand, M.H., 1995. Latin American women speak on development: Are we listening yet? *In*: Parpart, J.L. and Marchand, M. H., eds. *Feminism/ Postmodernism/ Development*. London/New York: Routledge, pp. 56-72.

Malinowski, B., 1922. *Argonauts of the Western Pacific: An Account of Native Enterprise and Adventure in the Melanesian New Guinea.* London: RKP.

Marshall, C. and Rossman, G.B., 1995. *Designing Qualitative Research.* California: Sage.

Mashman, V., 1991.Warriors and weavers: A study of gender relations among the Iban of Sarawak. *In:* Sutlive, V. H., ed. *Female and Male in Borneo: Contributions and Challenges to Gender Studies.* Shanghai, VA: Borneo Research Council Monograph, pp. 231-270. . Maseman, V.L., 1982. Critical ethnography in the study of comparative education, *Comparative Education Review*, February, 1-15.

Mascia-Lees, F. E., Sharpe, P. & Cohen, C. B. 1989. The postmodernist turn in anthropology: Cautions from a feminist perspective. *Signs,* 15, 7-33.

Mascia-Lees, F.E., Sharpe, P. and Cohen, C.B., 1989. The postmodernist turn in anthropology: Cautions from a feminist perspective'. *SIGNS, Journal of Women in Culture and Society.* 15 (1) Autumn, 7-33.

May, T., 1999. *Social Research: Issues, Methods and Process.* 2nd Edition. Buckingham: Open University Press.

Maynard, M., 1994. Methods, practice and epistemology: The debate about feminism and research. *In:* Maynard, M. and Purvis, J., ed. *Researching Women's Lives from a Feminist Perspective.* London: Taylor and Francis, pp. 10-26.

McCulloch, J., 2001. The theory and practice of European psychiatry in colonial Africa. *In:* Bhugra, D. and Littlewood, R., eds. *Colonialism and Psychiatry.* Oxford: Oxford University Press, pp. 76-104.

McGinty, R., 1996. Good stories and stereotypes. *In:* Read, J. and Reynolds, J., eds. *Speaking Our Minds: An Anthology of Personal Experiences of Mental Distress and Its Consequences,* Houndsmill, Basingstoke: The Open University/ MacMillan Press Ltd, pp. 91-94.

McLaughlin, L.A. and Braun, K.L, 1998. Asian and Pacific Islander cultural values: Considerations for health care decision making, *Health and Social Work.* 2 (2) May, 1-16.

McSherry, J., 1998. Spirituality: In pursuit of conceptual and theoretical unity, *Journal of Advanced Nursing.* 27 (4), 683-691.

Mead, M., 1943. *Coming of Age in Samoa.* Harmondsworth: Penguin.

Mental Health Act 2001, Act 615. Kuala Lumpur.

Mental Health Ordinance Sarawak, No 16 of 1961. Kuala Lumpur.

Mies, M., 1994. Towards a methodology for feminist research. *In:* Hammersley, M., ed. *Social Research: Philosophy, Politics and Practice.* London: The Open University/Sage Publications, pp. 64-82,

Miles, A., 1981. *The Mentally Ill in Contemporary Society.* Oxford: Martin Robertson.

Miles, M.B. and Huberman, M.A., 1994. *Qualitative Data Analysis*. Thousand Oaks/London: Sage Publications.

Mitchell, R.G. and Charmas, K., 1996. Telling tales, writing stories, *Journal of Contemporary Ethnograph*, 25 (1), 144-166.

Mo, G.-M., Chen, G.-Q., Li, L.-X. and Tseng, W.-S., 1995. Koro epidemic in Southern China. *In*: Tsung-Yi Lin, Wen-Shing Tseng and Eng-Kung Yeh., eds. *Chinese Societies and Mental Health*. Hong Kong: Oxford University Press, pp. 231-246.

Mohanty, C.T., 1991. Cartographies of struggle: Third World women and the politics of feminism. *In*: C. T. Mohanty, C.T., Russo, A. and Torres, L., eds. *Third World Women and the Politics of Feminism*. Bloomington/Indianapolis: Indiana University Press, pp. 1-50.

Monnig Atkinson, J., 1990. How gender makes a difference in Wana society. *In*: Monnig Atkinson, J. and Errington, S., eds. *Power & Difference: Gender in Island Southeast Asia*. Stanford California: Stanford University Press, pp. 59-93.

Montgomery, P., 2001. Shifting meaning of asylum. *Journal of Advanced Nursing*, 33(4), 425-431.

Moore, H.L., 1992. *Feminism and Anthropology*. Cambridge: Polity Press.

Murphy, E., 1991. *After the Asylums: Community care for people with mental illness*. London: Faber and Faber.

Murphy, H.B.M., 1971. The beginnings of psychiatric treatment in the Peninsula. *In*: Tan, E.-S. and Wagner, N.N., eds. *Psychological Problems and Treatment in Malaysia*. Kuala Lumpur: University of Malaya Press, pp. 14-18.

Murphy, H.B.M., 1973. History and the evolution of syndromes: The striking case of latah and amok. In: M. Hammer, M., Salzinger, K. and Sutton, S., eds. *Psychopathology: contributions from the social, behavioural, and biological sciences*. New York: Wiley, pp. 33-43.

Murphy, J.M., 1978. Culture and Mental Health. *Health and the Human Condition: Perspectives on Medical Anthropology*. In: Logan, M.H. and E.E. Hunt, E.E., eds Mass., USA: Duxbury Press, pp. 247-258.

Narayan, K., 1997. How Native is a 'Native' Anthropologist? *In*: L. Lamphere, L. and Ragoné, H, et al., eds. *Situated Lives: Gender and Culture in Everyday Life*. London/ New York: Routledge

Nazroo, J.Y., 1997. *Ethnicity and Mental Health*. London: Policy Studies Institute.

Nettle, M., 1996. Listening in the asylum. *In*: Read, J. and Reynolds, J., eds. *Speaking Our Minds: An Anthology of Personal Experiences of Mental Distress and Its Consequences*. Houndsmill, Basingstoke: The Open University/ MacMillan Press Ltd, pp. 202-206.

Ng, B.-Y. and Chee, K-T., 2006. A brief history of psychiatry in Singapore, *International Review of Psychiatry*, 18(4), 355-361.

Nichler, M., 1992. The Introduction. *In*: Nichler, M., ed. *Anthropological Approaches to the Study of Ethnomedicine*. Amersterdam: Gordon & Breech Scientific Publishers, pp. ix-.

Nieuwenhuis, A., 1929. Ten years of hygiene and ethnography in primitive Borneo (1891-1901). *In*: Schrieke, B. *The Effect of Western Influence on Native Civilizations in the Malay Archipelago*. Batavia: G. Kolff & Co.

Nissom, M.P. and Schmidt, K.E., 1967. Land-Dayak concept of mental illness, *The Medical Journal of Malaya*, XX1(4), 352-357.

Nolan, P. , 1997. Towards a rhetoric of spirituality in mental health care, *Journal of Advanced Nursing*, 26, 289-294.

Northrup, C., 1995. *Women's Bodies, Women's Wisdom*. USA/Canada: Bantam Books.

Oakley, A., 1984. Interviewing women: a contradiction in terms. Roberts, H., ed. *Doing Feminist Research*. London: Routledge and Kegan Paul, pp. 30-61.

O'Hagan, M., 1996. Two accounts of mental distress. *In*: Read, J. and Reynolds, J., eds. *Speaking Our Minds: An Anthology of Personal Experiences of Mental Distress and Its Consequences*. Houndsmill, Basingstoke: The Open University/ MacMillan Press Ltd, pp. 44-50.

Oldnall, A., 1996. A critical analysis of nursing: meeting the spiritual needs of patients, *Journal of Advanced Nursing*, 5 (2), 138-144.

Ong, A. (1995) 'State Versus Islam: Malay Families, Women's Bodies, and the Body Politic in Malaysia'. *In* : Onw, A. and Peletz, M.G., eds. *Bewitching Women, Pious Men: Gender and Body Politics in Southeast Asia*. Berkeley: University of California, pp.159-194.

Ong, A., 1990. Japanese factories, Malay workers: class and sexual metaphors in West Malaysia. *In*: Monnig Atkinson, J. and Errington, S., eds. *Power & Difference: Gender in Island Southeast Asia*. Stanford California: Stanford University Press, pp. 395-422

Orme, J., 1994. Violent women. *In*: Lupton, C. and Gillespie, T., eds. *Working with Violence*. Houndsmill, Basingstoke: Macmillan Press, pp. 170-189.

Ortner, S.B., 1995. Resistance and the Problem of Ethnographic Refusal, *Comparative Studies in Society and History*, 22 (1), 189-224.

Padmini Selvaratnam, D., 2001. The Malaysian Women's Role in Development, *The Third Malaysian Studies Conference*. UKM Bangi. 6-8th August

Pang, A.H.T., Yip, K.C., Cheung, H.K. and Yeung, O.C.Y., 1997. Community psychiatry in Hong Kong'. *The International Journal of Social Psychiatry*. 43 (3), 213 – 216.

Parpart, J. L. and Marchand, M.H., 1995. Exploding the cannon: An Introduction/ Conclusion. *In*: Parpart, J.L. and Marchand, M.H., eds. *Feminism Postmodernism Development*. London/New York: Routledge, pp. 1-22.

Parr, H, and Philo, C., 1996) 'A Forbidding Fortress of Locks, Bars and Padded Cells': *The locational history of mental health care in Nottingham*. Hisotrical Geography Research Series, Number 32.

Payne, M., 1995. *Social Work and Community Care*. Houndsmill, Basingstoke: Palgrave Macmillan.

Patai, D., 1991. U.S. Academics and Third World Women: Is Ethical Research Possible? *Women's Words: The Feminist Practice of Oral History*. NY/London: Routledge.

Pearson, G., 1993. Talking a good fight: Authenticity and distance in the ethnographer's craft. *In*: Hobbs, D. and May, T., eds. *Interpreting the Field, Accounts of Ethnography*. Oxford: Clarendon Press, pp. vii-xviiii.

Peletz, M.G. (1995) Neither reasonable nor responsible: Contrasting representations of masculinity in a Malay society' *In* : Onw, A. and Peletz, M.G., eds. *Bewitching Women, Pious Men: Gender and Body Politics in Southeast Asia*. Berkeley: University of California, pp.76-123. . Perkins, R., 1996. Choosing ECT. *In*: Read, J. and Reynolds, J., eds. *Speaking Our Minds: An Anthology of Personal Experiences of Mental Distress and Its Consequences'*. Houndsmill, Basingstoke: The Open University MacMillan Press Ltd, pp. 66-70.

Perutz, K., 1971. *Beyond the Looking Glass*. Penguin Books, Harmondsworth, Middlesex.

Pettman, J., 1992. *Living in the Margins: Racism, Sexism and Feminism in Australia*. Australia: Allen and Unwin.

Piddock, S., 2004. Possibilities and realities: South Australia's asylums in the 19th Century, *American Psychiatry*, 12(2), 172-175.

Pilgrim, D., 1988. British special hospitals. *In*: Ramon, S. and Giannichedda, M.G., eds. *Psychiatry in Transition: The British and Italian Experience*. London: Pluto Press

Pols, H., 2006. The development of psychiatry in Indonesia: From colonial to modern times. *International Review of Psychiatry*, 18(4), 363-370.

Porter, R., 2006, *Madmen*. Stroud, Glos: Tempus Publishing Limited.

Porter, R.,1983 The Rage of party: A glorious revolution of English psychiatry? *Medical History*, 27, 35-50.

Potter, R.B. and Phillips, J., 2006. 'Mad dogs and transnational migrants?' Bajan-Brits second-generation migrants and accusations of madness, *Annals of the Association of American Geographers*, 96(3), 586-600.

PNMB (1991). *Sixth Malaysia Plan*. Kuala Lumpur: PNMB.

PNMB (1993). *Mid Term Review of the Sixth Malaysia Plan*. Kuala Lumpur: PNMB.

PNMB (1996) Seventh Malaysia Plan 1996-2000, 89-96. Kuala Lumpur: PNMB.

Pringle, N.N. and Thompson, P.J., 1999. *Social Work, Psychiatry and the Law*. London: William Heineman Ltd.

Prior, L., 1993, *The Social Organisation of Mental Illness*. London: Sage Publishers.

Punch, M., 1994. Observation and the police: The research experience. *In*: Hammersley, M., ed. *Social Research: Philosophy, Politics and Practice*. London: The Open University/Sage Publications, pp. 181-199.

Purcell, V., 1948. *The Chinese in Malaya*. London: Oxford University Press.

Quantz, R.A., 1992. On critical ethnography with some postmodern considerations. *In*: in M. D. LeCompte, M.D., Millroy, W.L. and Preissle, J., eds. *The Handbook of Qualitative Research in Education*. San Diego: Academic Press, pp. 447-506.

Rack, P., 1982. *Race, Culture and Mental Disorder*. London/New York: Tavistock.

Ramon, S. 1988. Introduction. *In*: Ramon, S. and Giannichedda, M.G., eds. *Psychiatry in* Transition: The British and Italian Experience. London: Pluto Press.

Ramon, S., 1996. *Mental Health in Europe: Ends, Beginnings and Rediscoveries*. Houndsmill, Basingstoke: MacMillan Press Ltd/MIND Publications.

Razali, S.M., 1995. Psychiatrists and folk healers in Malaysia, *World Health Forum*, 16, 56-58.

Razali, S.M., Khan, U. And Hasanah, C., 1996. Belief in supernatural causes of mental illness among Malay patients: impact on treatment, *ACTA Psychiatrica Scandinavica*. 94: 229-233.

Razali, S.M., 1997. Legitimising Traditional Medicine: A Personal View, *Malaysian Psychiatry*, 3 (3/4), 72-74.

Redfield Jamison, K., 1997. *An Unquiet Mind*. London: Picador.

Reece, R.H.W., 1991. European-indigenous miscegenation and social status in nineteenth Century Borneo. *In*: Sutlive, V. H., ed. *Female and Male in Borneo: Contributions and Challenges to Gender Studies*. Shanghai, VA: Borneo Research Council Monograph, pp. 455-488.

Report of the Mental Health Nursing Review Team, 1994. *Working in Partnership*. London: Department of Health, HMSO.

Rhi, B.Y., Ha, K.S., Kim, Y.S., Sasaki, Y., Young, D., Wood, T.-H., Laraya, L.T., and Yanchun, Y., 1995.The Health care seeking behavior of schizophrenic patients in 6 East Asian Areas, *International Journal of Social Psychiatry*, 41 (3), 190-209.

Roberts, H., 1984. Women and their doctors: power and powerlessness in the research process. *In*: Roberts, H., ed. *Doing Feminist Research*. London: Routledge and Kegan Paul, pp. 7-29.

Rogers, A. and Pilgrim, D., 1992. Service users views of psychiatric nurses, *British Journal of Nursing*, 3 (1), 16-18.

Rogers, A., Pilgrim, D. and Lacey, R., 1993. *Experiencing Psychiatry: Users' Views of Services*. London: MacMillan Press/MIND Publications.

Romanucci-Ross, L., 1997a. The 'new psychiatry': From ideology to cultural error. *In*: Romanucci-Ross, L., Moerman, D.E. and Tancredi, L.R., eds. *The Anthropology of Medicine: From Culture to Method*. Westport, Connecticut/London: Bergin & Garvey, pp. 318-335.

Romanucci-Ross, L., 1997b. The impassioned knowledge of the Shaman. *In*: Romanucci-Ross, L., Moerman, D.E. and Tancredi, L.R., eds. *The Anthropology of Medicine: From Culture to Method*. Westport, Connecticut/London: Bergin & Garvey, pp. 215-223.

Rosenhan, D.L., 1993. On Being Sane in insane places. *In*: Pontell, H.N., ed. *Social Deviance: Readings in Theory and Research*. New Jersey: Prentice-Hall Inc.

Rostom, M. and Lee, S., 1996. *Mental Health Services in Malaysia: Report of a StudyTour*. Hertfordshire: University of Hertfordshire.

Rousseau, J., 1993. From shamans to priests: Towards the professionalization of religious specialists among the Kayan. *In*: Winzeler, R.L., ed. (Ed) *The Seen and the Unseen: Shamanism, Mediumship and Possession in Borneo*. Virginia, USA: Ashley Printing Services, pp. 131-150.

Rousseau, J., 1991. Gender and Class in Central Borneo. *In*: V. H. Sutlive, V.H., ed. *Female and Male in Borneo: Contributions and Challenges to Gender Studies*. Virginia, Borneo Research Council Monograph, Inc, pp. 403-414.

Rowett, C. and Vaughan P. J., 1981. Women and Broadmoor: Treatment and control in a special hospital. *In*: Hutter, B. and Williams, G., eds. *Controlling Women, the Normal and the Deviant*. London/Oxford: Croom Helm, pp. 131-153.

Russell, D., 1995. *Women, Madness and Medicine*. Cambridge: Polity Press.

Rutherford, S., 2008. *The Victorian Asylum*. Oxford: Shire Library.

Sacks, O., 1995. An Anthropologist on Mars. London: Pan Books.

Sadowsky, J., 2003, The social world and the reality of mental illness: Lessons from colonial psychiatry, *Harvard Review of Psychiatry*, 11, 210-214.

Sadowsky, J., 1999. *Imperial Bedlam: Institutions of madness in colonial Southwest Nigeria*. Berkeley: University of California Press.

Sainsbury Centre for Mental Health, 1998. *Acute Problems: A Survey of the quality of care in acute psychiatric wards*. London: The Sainsbury Centre.

Saris, J. A., 1996. Mad kings, proper houses and an asylum in rural Ireland, *American Anthropologist*, 98 (3), 539 -554.

Sartorius, N., Jablensky, A. and Shapiro, R., 1977. Two-year follow-up of the patients included in the WHO International Pilot Study of Schizophrenia, *Psychological Medicine*. 7, 529-541.

Sashidharan, S.P. and Francis, F., 1993. Epidemiology, ethnicity and schizophrenia. *In*: Ahmad,W. I.U., ed. *'Race' and Health in Contemporary Britain*. Buckingham: Open University Press, pp. 113-129.

Savage, C., Leighton, A.H. and Leighton, D.C., 1966. The Problem of Cross-Cultural Identification of Psychiatric Disorders. *In*: Murphy, H.M. and Leighton, A.H., eds. *Approaches to Cross Cultural Psychiatry*: Ithaca, New York: Cornell University Press, pp. 4-

Scheff, T.J., 1966. *Being Mentally Ill: A Sociological Theory*. New York: Aldine Publishing Company. *In*: Heller, T., Reynolds, J., Gomm, R., Muston, R. and Pattison, S. eds. *Mental Health Matters*. Houndsmill, Basingstoke. The Open University/Macmillan, pp. 64-69.

Scheff, T. J., 1996. Labelling mental illness. *In*: Heller, T., Reynolds, J., Gomm, R., Muston, R. and Pattison, S. eds. *Mental Health Matters*. Houndsmill, Basingstoke. The Open University/Macmillan, p. 64-69.

Scheper-Hughes, N., 1979. *Saints, Scholars and Schizophrenics: Mental Illness in Rural Ireland*. Berkeley and Los Angeles: University of California Press.

Scheper-Hughes, N., 1992. *Death Without Weeping*. Berkeley: University of California Press.

Scheper-Hughes, N. and Lovell, A.M., 1986. Breaking the circuit of social control: Lessons in public psychiatry from Italy and Franco Basaglia, *Social Science and Medicine*, 23 (2), 159-178.

Schmidt, K.E., 1961. Management of schizophrenia in Sarawak Mental Hospital, 1959, *Journal of Mental Science*, 107, 157-160.

Schmidt, K.E., 1964. Folk psychiatry in Sarawak: A tentative system of psychiatry in the Iban. *In*: Kiev, A., ed. *Magic, Faith and Healing*. New York: The Free Press, pp. 139-

Schneider, W.M. and Schneider, M., 1991. Male/female distinction among the Selako. *In*: Sutlive, V. H., ed. *Female and Male in Borneo: Contributions and Challenges to Gender Studies*. Shanghai, VA: Borneo Research Council Monograph, pp. 345-364.

Scull, A.T., 1979. *Museums of Madness*. Middlesex, UK: Penguin.

Scull, A., 1993. *The Most Solitary of Afflictions: Madness and Society in Britain, 1700- 1900*. New Haven: Yale University Press.

Selig, N., 1988. Ethnicity and gender as uncomfortable issues. *In*: Ramon, S. and Giannichedda, M.G., eds. *Psychiatry in Transition: The British and Italian Experience*. London: Pluto Press, pp. 90-98.

Soja, E., 1996. *Thirdspace*. Oxford: Blackwell.

Standing Nursing and Midwifery Advisory Committee (SNMAC), 1999. *Mental Health Nursing: 'Addressing Acute Concerns'*. London: Department of Health.

Stanley, L. and Wise, S., 1993. *Breaking Out Again: Feminist Ontology and Epistemology*. London/New York: Routledge.

Strathern, M., 1987. An awkward relationship: The case of feminism and anthropology, *Signs: Journal of Women in Culture and Society*, 12(2), 276-292.

Stoler, L., 1991. Carnal knowledge and imperial power: Gender, race, and morality in Colonial Asia. *In*: M. di Leonardo, M., ed. *Gender at the Crossroads of Knowledge: Feminist Anthropology in the Postmodern Era*. California: Berkeley, pp. 51-101.

Shaffir, W.B., 1991. Managing a convincing self-presentation: some personal reflections on entering the field. *In*: Shaffir, W.B. and Stebbins, R. A., eds. *Experiencing Fieldwork*. Newbury Park, C.A./ London: Sage Publications, pp. 72-82.

Shorter, E., 1997. *A History of Psychiatry*. New York: John Wiley & Sons.

Showalter, E., 1981. Victorian women and insanity. *In*: Scull, A., ed. *Madhouses, Mad Doctors and Madmen*. London: The Athlone Press, pp. 313-331.

Showalter, E., 1985. *The Female Malady: Women, Madness and English Culture 1830- 1980*. London: Virago Press.

Silverman, D., 1993. *Interpreting Qualitative Data*. London/Thousand Oaks: Sage Publications.

Silverman, J., 1967. Shamans and acute schizophrenia, *American Anthropologist*, 69, 21-31.

Simon, R.I. and Dippo, D. , 1986. On critical ethnographic work, *Anthropology and Education Quarterly*, 17, 185-202.

Simons, R.C., 1996. *Boo! Culture, Experience and the Startle Reflex*. New York: Oxford University Press.

Sindzingre, N., 1995. The need for meaning: The explanations of ill fortune among the Senufo. *In*: Augé, M. and Herzlich, C., eds. *The Meaning of Illness: Anthropology & History of Sociology*. Luxembourg: Harwood Academic Publisher, pp. 71-96.

Spiro, M.E. and D'Andrade, R., 1967. A cross-cultural study of some supernatural beliefs. *In*: C. S. Ford, C.S., ed. *Cross-Cultural Approaches*. Newhaven: HRAF Press.

Spores, J.C., 1988. *Running Amok: An Historical Inquiry*. Ohio: Ohio University Press.

Spradley, J.P., 1980. *Participant Observation*. Florida: Harcourt Brace Jovanovitch College Publishers.

Spradley, J.P., 1979. *The Ethnographic Interview*. Florida: Harcourt Brace Jovanovitch College Publishers.

Stacey, J. (1991) 'Can There Be a Feminist Ethnography?', in S. Berger Gluck and D. Patai (Eds) *Women's Words. The Feminist Practice of Oral History* London/ New York: Routledge.

Stanley, L. and Wise, S. (1993) *Breaking Out Again: Feminist Ontology and Epistemology*. London/New York: Routledge.

Strutti, C. and Rauber, S., 1994. Leros and the Greek Mental Health System'. *International Journal of Social Psychiatry*, 40 (4), 306-312.

Sundberg, N.D., Hadiyono, J.P., Latkin, C.A. and Padilla, J., 1995. Cross-cultural prevention program transfer: Questions regarding developing countries. *The Journal of Primary Prevention*. 15 (4): 361-376.

Sutlive, C. and Appell, G.N., 1991. Introduction. *In:*. Sutlive,V. H, ed. *Female and Male in Borneo: Contributions and Challenges to Gender Studies*. Virginia, Borneo Research Council Monograph, Inc., pp.vii- xivi

Sutlive, V., 1991. Keling and kumang in town: urban migration and differential effects on Iban women and men. *In:* Sutlive, V. H., ed. *Female and Male in Borneo: Contributions and Challenges to Gender Studies*. Shanghai, VA: Borneo Research Council Monograph, pp. 489-528.

Sutton, J.R., 1991. The political economy of madness: the expansion of the asylum in progressive America, *American Sociological Review*, 56, 665-678.

Swettenham, F. , 1906. *British Malaya*. London: George Allen & Unwin, Ltd.

Szasz, T., 1994. Psychiatric diagnosis, psychiatric power and psychiatric abuse, *Journal of Medical Ethics*, 20, 135 - 138.

Szasz, T.S., 1974. *The Myth of Mental Illness*. New York: Harper & Row.

Tan, E.-S. and Wagner, N.N. (1971) Psychiatry in Malaysia. *In:* Tan, E.-S. N. N. Wagner, N.N., eds. *Psychological Problems and Treatment in Malaysia*. Kuala Lumpur: University of Malaya Press, pp. 1-13.

Tang, M. and Cuninghame, C., 1996. Focusing on health: focus groups for consulting about health needs. *In:* Heller, T., Reynolds, J., Gomm, R., Muston, R. and Pattison, S. eds. *Mental Health Matters*. Houndsmill, Basingstoke. The Open University/Macmillan, pp. 260-266.

Taylor, L., 1996. ECT is Barbaric. *In:* Read, J. and Reynolds, J., eds. *Speaking Our Minds: An Anthology of Personal Experiences of Mental Distress and Its Consequences'*. Houndsmill, Basingstoke: The Open University MacMillan Press Ltd, 63-65.

Taylor, S.J., 1991. Leaving the field: Research, relationships and responsibilities. *In:* Shaffir, W.B. and Stebbins, R. A., eds. *Experiencing Fieldwork*. Newbury Park, C.A./ London: Sage Publications, pp. 238-247.

Teoh, J.I., 1971. History of institutional psychiatric care in Singapore 1862-1967. *In:* Tan, E.-S. and Wagner, N.N., eds. *Psychological Problems and Treatment in Malaysia*. Kuala Lumpur: University of Malaya Press, pp.19-30.

Terrell. D., 1994. Abnormal psychology. *In:* Matsumo, D., ed. *People: Psychology from a Cultural Perspective*. California: Brooks/Cole Publishing Co., pp. 138-156.

Tesch, R., 1991. Software for qualitative researchers: Analysis needs and program Capabilities. *In:* Lee, R.M. and Fielding, N.G., eds. *Using Computers in Qualitative Research*. London, Newbury Park, C.A.: Sage Publications, pp. 16-37.

The Mental Health Act Commission, 1997. *The National Visit*. London: Sainsbury Centre for Mental Health.

Thomas, J. , 1983. Toward a Critical Ethnography, *Urban Life*, 11 (4), 477- 490.

Thompson, N., 1997. *Anti-Discriminatory Practice*. 2nd Edition. Basingstoke: BASW/MacMillan Press.

Trad, P.V., 1991. The Ultimate stigma of mental illness, *American Journal of Psychotherapy*, 45 (4), 463-467.

Turner, B., 1981. Some practical aspects of qualitative data analysis: One way of organising the cognitive processes associated with the generation of grounded theory. *Quality and Quantity*, 15, 225-6.

Turner, B.S. , 1992. *Medical Power and Social Knowledge*. London: Sage Publications.

Ussher, J., 1991. *Women's Madness: Misogyny or Mental Illness*. New York: Harvester Wheatsheaf.

Valeri, V., 1990. Both nature and culture. Reflections on menstrual and parturitional Taboos in Huaulu, Seram. *In*: Monnig Atkinson, J. and Errington, S., eds. *Power & Difference: Gender in Island Southeast Asia*. Stanford California: Stanford University Press, pp. 235-272.

Vanchieri, C., 1995. Cultural gaps leave patients angry, doctors confused, *Journal of the National Cancer Institute*, 87 (21), 15-18.

Van Maanen, J., 1988. *Tales of the Field: On Writing Ethnography*. Chicago: University of Chicago.

Van Maanen, J., 1991. Playing back the tape: Early days in the field. *In*: Shaffir, W.B. and Stebbins, R. A., eds. *Experiencing Fieldwork*. Newbury Park, C.A./London: Sage Publications, pp. 31-42.

Vaughan, M., 2007. Introduction. *In*: Mahone, S. and Vaughan, M., eds. *Psychiatry and Empire*. Houndsmill, Basingstoke: Palgrave Macmillan, pp. 1-16.

Visweswaran, K., 1998. Defining feminist ethnography. *Inscriptions*, 3 (4), 27-44.

Wagner. W., Duveen, G., Themel, M. and Verma, J., 1999. The modernization of tradition: Thinking about madness in Patna, India. *Culture & Psychology*, 5(4), 413-445.

Walsh, R., 1994. The making of a shaman, *Journal of Humanistic Psychology*, 34 (3) Summer, 7-24.

Warner, R., 1996. The cultural context of mental distress. *In*: Heller, T., Reynolds, J., Gomm, R., Muston, R. and Pattison, S. eds. *Mental Health Matters*. Houndsmill, Basingstoke. The Open University/Macmillan, pp. 54-63.

Warren, C.A.B., 1988. *Gender Issues in Field Research*. Newbury Park, California: Sage Publications.

Waxler, N.E., 1977. Is mental illness cured in traditional societies? A theoretical analysis, *Culture, Medicine and Psychiatry* 1, 233- 253.

Wessels, W.H., 1985. The traditional healer and psychiatry. *Australian and New Zealand Journal of Psychiatry*, 19, 283-286.

Wetzel, J.W., 2000. Women and mental health: a global perspective. *International Social Work*, 43 (2) April, 205-215.

Wikan, U., 1993. Beyond the words: The power of resonance. *In*: Pálsson, G., ed. *Beyond Boundaries*. Oxford: Berg Publishing Ltd, pp. 184-210.

Williams, J., 1999. Social inequalities and mental health. *In*: Newnes, C. and Holmes, G., eds. *This is Madness: A Critical Look at Psychiatry and Mental Health Services*. Ross-on-Wye: PCCS Books.

Wintersteen, R.T. et al. (1997) 'Families and mental illness: observations from two developing countries'. *International Social Work*. 40: 191-207.

Winzeler, R.L., 1995. *Latah in Southeast Asia: The History and Ethnography of a Culture-Bound Syndrome*. Cambridge: Cambridge University Press.

Witz, A., 1992. *Professions and Patriarchy*. London: Routledge.

Woon, T.-H., 1971. Central Mental Hospital, Tanjong Rambutan. *In*: Tan, E.-S. and Wagner, N.N., eds. *Psychological Problems and Treatment in Malaysia*. Kuala Lumpur: University of Malaya Press, pp. 31-47.

Yee, L. and Shun Au., 1997. *Chinese Mental Health Issues in Britain*. London: Mental Health Foundation.

Yee, M. (2001) Women transmigrants in Malaysia: Identity, work and the household. *The Third Malaysian Studies Conference*. UKM Bangi. 6-8th August.

Yip, K-S. (2005) An historical review of the Mental Health Services in the People's Republic of China'. *International Journal of Social Psychiatry*, 51, 106-117.

Younger, J. (1995) 'The alienation of the sufferer'. *Advances in Nursing Science*, 17 (4), 53-72.

Index

Asian migrant labour 48, 50
Asian women 42, 149, 200
assaults see sexual abuse; violence
asylums
    dehumanisation 6, 163, 164
    England 31–5, 38, 49, 164
    historical perspective in Europe 31–5, 38
    historical perspective in the American colonies 34
    history of psychiatry/colonial psychiatry 37–8
    locked ward policies 162, 163–4, 168–9
    Malaya 48–51, 53
    multiculturalism in Malaysia 153
    negative connotations 4, 5–6
    North America 49
    open ward policies 161–2, 164–5
    as refuge/retreat 4, 80, 123, 124, 142, 175, 199, 200
    terminology 4
    therapeutic aspects 65
Atkinson, J.M. 113, 139
Atkinson, P. 11
Au, S. 54, 157
Aull Davies, C. 12, 26
Aunger, R. 11
awakenings 20, 120

Baba, I. 5, 41, 48, 66, 148, 149, 153, 187, 188
badminton 85, 143, 146
Bahasa Malayu language 26–7, 28, 118
Bailey, C.A. 23
Baker, A.A. 85
Bannister, P. 20
Barham, P. 32, 34, 96, 110, 120, 193
Barnes, M. 51, 52, 53, 81, 155, 180, 183
Barrett, R.J. 25, 188
barter, by patients 89, 100, 101–2, 105, 107–8, 137
Basagalia, Franco 6, 161
basket weaving 113, 114
Battie, William 32
Beasley, C. 140
beauty sessions 146–8, 200

children 42, 81, 82
China 39–40
Chinese families 156, 157–8
Chinese languages 26, 27
Chinese men 156
Chinese migrant workers 41, 50, 156–7, 158
Chinese nursing staff 159
Chinese patients
 Britain 54
 ethnic typecasting and racism by staff 156–8, 159, 201
 Malaysia 153, 154, 155
 medical assessment, public knowledge 118
 predominance in Hospital Tranquillity 89, 153, 154
 see also Chua (male Chinese patient); Foo (male Chinese patient); Jacob (male Chinese patient); Margo (female Chinese patient); Maria (female Chinese patient); Patrick (male Chinese patient); Tan Siew (male Chinese patient); Teo (male Chinese patient); Wei Hua (female Chinese patient)
Chinese people 5, 157, 158, 159
Chinese staff 156, 157, 159
Chinese traditional healers 126
Chong, G. 64–5, 78, 128, 175, 176, 177, 179, 182
chores/tasks of patients
 caring tasks 111–12, 200
 daily routines 87
 rewarding 'prominent' patients 104, 105, 107, 109, 110
Christianity
 acceptance of ECT 132
 asylums in Europe 32
 Borneo 56
 Malaysia 155
 spirituality and healing 123–4, 125
 tolerance of mental illness 158
 women's chastity 139
'chronic' patients
 Britain 74
 Chinese predominance 154, 155, 157
 concept 71–5
 discharge, impossibility of 82–3
chronic wards
 described 71–2, 75

ECT (electro-convulsive therapy), attitudes towards 130
   fear of patients and risk of violence 167, 171–2
   hierarchies 172
   language usage 28
   medical assessment, public knowledge 118
   medical assistants/nursing staff professional standards, opinions about 194–5
   medical/psychiatric training 45, 46–7, 65, 124, 194
   non-commitment towards psychiatry 190, 191–2, 195
   occupational therapy 115
   private general practice 191, 195
   see also psychiatrists
dominant ward relationships 103–10
dominant ward relationships, failure to attain/demotion from 108–9, 110
Down's Syndrome 77, 109
dukan (traditional healer) 106–7, 123–4
Dutch colonialism 35, 36, 56–63

earnings of patients 110, 114, 115, 116
Eaton, P. 5, 41
economic exploitation
   colonialism 4, 41, 61
   labour of patients 110, 116, 200
   by migrant workers 61, 157
ECT (electro-convulsive therapy)
   asylums in Malaya 55
   Britain 129
   and class 191
   control by staff 129–33, 164, 201
   negative connotations of psychiatric hospitals 6
Edward (male patient) 124
elderly female patients 140, 143–4, 147
Ellis, William Gilmore see Gilmore Ellis, William
Elvis (male Bidayuh patient) 102, 165
Elynna (female Iban patient) 81–2
emancipatory ethnography 11–13
emasculation 80, 156
emotional support 96, 97, 111, 188
empathy, planning the research 22, 27–8
England
   asylums 31–5, 38, 49, 91, 161, 164

Female Ward 1
  bed sharing 86–7
  daily routines 87, 88
  dominant relationships 105–6
  ECT (electro-convulsive therapy) 129, 132–3
  escorted discharge rules 83–4
  ethnic typecasting and racism by nursing staff 158
  ethnicity of patients 154
  fear of patients by researcher 171
  Field notes 83–4, 91, 92–3, 118, 129, 136–7, 141
  food 90
  locked section of ward 109, 136–7, 138, 144–5
  locked wards 85
  medical assessment, public knowledge 118
  medication 119
  mothers 81, 141–2
  open wards 141
  physical restraints 144–5
  planning the research 19
  reciprocal relationships 97–8
  recreation 146, 148
  restriction of freedom 139
  sexuality 140–1, 142, 149–51
  spatial layout and appearance 85
  uniforms 91, 92–4
Female Ward 2
  'chronic' patients 72
  dominant relationships 104, 105
  ethnicity of patients 154
  familial relationships 111–12
  Field notes 17–18, 72, 104, 111–12, 147
  hostility towards researcher 17–18
  locked section of ward 105
  locked wards 85
  planning the research 19
  reciprocal relationships 101
  recreation 146, 147
  spatial layout and appearance 85–6
  violence 104–5
feminine pathology 51, 52

Howard, N.C. 123
Huberman, M.A. 15
Hughes, N. Scheper- see Scheper-Hughes, N.
Hui Ling, Miss (male transsexual patient) 16, 100, 148
humanitarianism 62, 175
husbands 82
hygiene deficiencies 87, 136, 162, 163, 164

Iban language 26–7
Iban patients 81–2, 156
Iban senior nursing staff 17–18
Iban traditional healers 58–9, 106, 126–7
ideal asylum 33–4, 69
illness, meanings 127
imprisonment, asylum concept 4
in-depth, unstructured interviews 10, 20–1
indefinite admissions 78, 79–80
Independence 41, 47
India 54, 125
    see also colonial India
Indian migrant workers 41, 50, 53, 153
Indian patients 155
indigenous people 5, 38, 39
individual interviews 10
Indonesia 35, 47, 111
Indonesia people 160
informal gatekeepers 14–18
institutionalisation, 'chronic' patients 73, 74, 75
institutionalised racism 53, 155, 159
institutionalised sexism 185
interpreters/translators 26, 27
intolerance of mental illness
    communities 96, 97
    families 35, 73, 74, 79–80, 96, 97, 189, 199
        Chinese families 156, 157–8
invisibility, observations in planning the research 20
'irredeemable' patients, 'chronic' patients 73–5
Islam
    bumiputera 5, 155
    ethnic typecasting 160

mental disorder classification in Malaya 43–4, 50

military regimentation 183

occupational therapy 114–15

open wards 138, 162

reciprocal relationships 22–3, 96, 97, 98

recreation 143, 146

restrictions on movement 85, 138, 162

sexuality 24, 143, 148

uniforms 92

violence 156, 165, 169–70

Male Ward 1

admissions 79

conflict 102

counselling, lack of 188

daily routines 87–8

dominant relationships 107

dominant relationships, failure to attain 108–9

ECT (electro-convulsive therapy) 131, 132

ethnicity of patients 154

familial relationships 110

Field notes 16–17, 89, 102, 108, 131, 136, 182

hostility 16–17

locked section of ward 119, 121, 131, 135–6, 137

mealtimes 89

medication 119, 120, 121

occupational therapy 114–15

planning the research 19

reciprocal relationships 96, 97, 98, 100

restrictions on movement 162

single males 81

spatial layout and appearance 85, 86

working conditions 182

Male Ward 2

dominant relationships 107–8

ethnicity of patients 154

Field notes 183

locked section of ward 85

locked wards 85

military regimentation of ward 183

planning the research 19

reciprocal relationships 101

Ong, A. 41, 42–3, 57, 112, 113
open wards
    appearance 86, 162
    England and Italy 161
    female patients 138, 141–2, 162
    male patients 138, 162
    policies 161–2, 164–5
    staff attitudes 161–2, 164, 201
    see also freedom of movement; locked wards; restriction of movement
opium use 49, 50
opportunism 138, 140, 168
opportunistic sampling 22
oppression
    ethnographic approach 12
    history of psychiatry/colonial psychiatry 38, 39
    labelling of mental illness 79
    migrant workers 155
    women 52–3, 82
orang buat (witch/sorcerer) 105–6, 128
orang gila (mad person) 96, 128
orang puteh (white person) 21, 148
Orme, J. 105, 165
Ortner, S.B. 11–12
'otherness' 45, 158
outpatients 118–19
overcrowding
    asylums, historical perspective in England and British Empire 34, 38, 164
    ECT and control 130, 201
    locked section of wards 85, 136
    public wards 70
overt observation 19–20

P., Dr. (female) 171
P., Nurse 83–4
Pang, A.H.T. 188
paranoid schizophrenia 107, 119
Parr, H. 71
participants 4, 14, 15–16
    see also directors of Hospital Tranquillity; patients; staff
passivity
    ethnic typecasting 156

locked wards 163
from patients towards staff 163, 169–73
reduction, effects of open wards 162, 164
from staff 164, 165, 166
ward relationships 101–2, 103, 104–5, 115–16
see also aggression; fear of patients' behaviour; risk of violence; sexual abuse
Visweswaran, K. 13
voluntary admissions 78
vulnerability, feminine stereotypes 139, 140–1, 142

Wagner, N.N. 48, 49, 51, 53, 63, 64, 155
Wagner, W. 125
ward life 79, 85–94, 136, 162, 163–4, 183–4, 198
ward relationships see conflict; dominant ward relationships; familial ward relationships; reciprocal ward relationships
wards see acute wards; Bunga Raya Ward; chronic wards; Female Ward 1; Female Ward 2; First-Class Ward; living conditions on wards; locked section of wards; locked wards; Male Ward 1; Male Ward 2; Male Ward 3; open wards; private wards; public wards; Second-Class Ward; ward life
warfare 61, 62
Warner, R. 59, 128
Waxler, N.E. 127–8
Wei Hua (female Chinese patient) 86–7, 144–5
Weng, Sister 168
Western ethnocentrism, colonial psychiatry and anthropology 45–7, 54, 65–6
Western health care 60, 62, 124–5, 175–6, 199
Western psychiatric training 45, 46–7, 65, 124, 194
Wetzel, J.W. 6, 52, 53, 76, 115
white ethnicity of researcher 2, 21, 148
wholeness, spirituality and healing 124
Wikan, U. 27
Williams, J. 52
Winzeler, R.L. 42, 43, 44, 106
witch/sorcerer (orang buat) 105–6, 128
withdrawal of researcher from research study 13, 203
Witz, A. 54, 115, 181
women
chastity 139–40, 141, 142
oppression 52–3, 82
psychoanalysis and anthropology 42
sexual abuse of 52, 139, 142